Critical Acclaim for the First Edition of

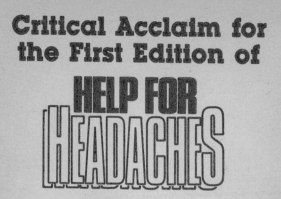

HELP FOR HEADACHES

W9-AYY-494

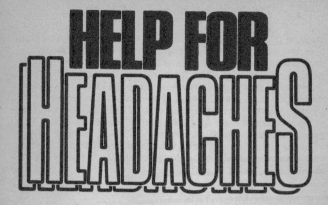

HELP FOR HEADACHES

adapted from *Headache Disorders*

JOEL R. SAPER, M.D., F.A.C.P.

WARNER BOOKS

A Warner Communications Company

WARNER BOOKS EDITION

Adaptation copyright © 1987 by Warner Books, Inc.
Copyright © 1983 by John Wright • PSG Inc.
All rights reserved. No part of this publication may be reproduced or transmitted in any form or by any means, electronic or mechanical, including photocopy, recording, or any information storage or retrieval system, without permission in writing from the publisher.

This Warner Books Edition is published by arrangement with PSG Publishing Company, Inc., 545 Great Road, Littleton, Massachusetts 01460

Cover design by Anthony Russo

Warner Books, Inc.
666 Fifth Avenue
New York, N.Y. 10103

A Warner Communications Company

Printed in the United States of America

First Warner Books Printing: August, 1987

10 9 8 7 6 5 4 3

To Renée, Lisa, Justin and Lauren
For their love, encouragement,
and very special patience

To my mother
For the spirit of compassion and so much more

Contents

About the Author

oel R. Saper, M.D., F.A.C.P., is the Director of the Michi-
an Headache and Neurological Institute in Ann Arbor,
lichigan, which he founded in 1978. This institute is the
rst comprehensive headache treatment and research center
a the world. In 1979 Dr. Saper and his colleagues developed
ae first inpatient (hospital) headache unit to serve patients
ith severe and intractable headache pain, and recently this
nit has been awarded the first national accreditation ever
iven to a headache treatment facility. Currently, the Insti-
ate is considered a leader in the treatment and research of
ead and neck pain, and patients from around the world are
eferred to it.

Dr. Saper became interested in head pain disorders while
erving as an assistant professor of neurology at the Univer-
ity of Michigan. In 1978 Dr. Saper left the University to
evelop the Institute and at that time became clinical associ-
te professor of medicine (neurology) at Michigan State
niversity.

In addition to his role in the Institute, Dr. Saper is a prolific writer and is currently working on his fifth medical book. Among his other books on the subjects of pain and neurology is *Freedom from Headaches*, originally published by Simon and Schuster and subsequently published in soft cover form by Fireside Press. This book is also the choice of *Consumer Reports*, which publishes *Freedom from Headaches* under its own imprint.

In addition, Dr. Saper is the Editor-in-Chief and primary author of *Topics in Pain Management*, an international newsletter on pain management therapy, and has written numerous articles and chapters for medical journals and books on headache and pain treatment and research. He speaks throughout the country to medical groups, major medical institutions, colleges, and to the public on subjects ranging from pain and its treatment to the changing role of medicine in our society. He is an officer and member of the Board of Directors of the American Association for the Study of Headache and a member of important committees for the American Association for Pain Medicine. Dr. Saper is a member of the American Pain Society, the American Epilepsy Society, the American Academy of Neurology, and numerous other medical groups.

Dr. Saper has been an invited guest on numerous regional and national television and radio programs, including ABC TV's *Nightline* with Ted Koppel, NBC Network News, and National Public Radio, and he is a regular guest on local talk shows, including WJR (Warren Pierce) and WXYZ (Mark Scott).

Dr. Saper is 43 years old and was born and raised in Joliet, Illinois. He received his Bachelor's Degree in history at the University of Wisconsin, his Medical Degree at the University of Illinois College of Medicine, and his neurological training at the University of Michigan. He is the father of three children aged 7, 5, and 4, and has lived in Ann Arbor since 1970.

ACKNOWLEDGMENTS

To Grace Lobel
For her profound understanding, friendship,
and endless energy on my behalf

To Jane Howard, my transcriptionist,
Whose extraordinary talent and endurance
have made this and
so many other projects possible

To Lillian Rodberg, The Manuscript Doctor,
Who edited the manuscript and translated
medical terms with the needs
of the lay reader continually in mind

SPECIAL ACKNOWLEDGMENT

To my Patients

For all that you have taught me
through your pain and perseverance,
and for the trust and inspiration
which continue to mean so much

CONTRIBUTORS

Michael R. Barnat, Ph.D., Licensed Psychologist, Senior Clinical Psychologist, Michigan Headache and Neurological Institute, P.C., Ann Arbor

Alvin E. Lake III, Ph.D., Licensed Psychologist, Senior Behavioral Psychologist, Coordinator of Psychophysiological Services, Michigan Headache and Neurological Institute, P.C., Ann Arbor

William G. Speed III, M.D., Associate Professor of Medicine, Johns Hopkins Hospital, Baltimore

1

Headache: The Problem

Headache is one of the most common of human afflictions. A recent Harris Poll commissioned by a drug manufacturer suggests that over 70% of U.S. households had individuals who experienced headaches. This means that 50 to 70 million Americans experience recurring headaches, which may account for more missed work and more visits to physicians than any other condition. Headache strikes rich and famous, educated and noneducated, young and old, and people of all geographic locations.

Most people who suffer from chronic headache are essentially healthy, but for many of them, attacks of headache become increasingly troublesome. Eventually, pain and its many complications will eventually affect the very fiber and quality of life. Even discriminating individuals are driven to seek a wide variety of treatments, many of which are frightening and painful. Sinus surgery, neck traction, hormone regulation, allergy desensitization, tooth extractions, hysterectomy, psychotherapy, hypnotism, chiropractic manipulation, and jaw reconstruction are but some of the techniques headache sufferers and their physicians have encountered in seeking relief.

Despite the staggering number of people who experience recurring headache, myth, misinformation, and mistreatment continue to surround this problem. Moreover, the medical approach to headaches and attitudes toward those who have them have not, until recently, kept pace with advances in modern science. Indeed, formal training in the treatment of pain has been historically absent from even the finest medical schools. Many otherwise qualified physicians readily admit that their approach to chronic headache is founded on traditional assumptions and at times prejudice.

Understandably, headache victims become confused and frustrated. The void created by the lack of concise and satisfactory scientific explanation and treatment leaves ample room for misunderstanding, improper treatment, and outright quackery. With this situation in mind, I have written this book. The facts and opinions presented here may enhance your understanding of this widespread yet inadequately treated condition.

Some Facts About Headaches

Did you know that an estimated 50 *million* pounds of aspirin—much of it for the relief of headache—are taken in the United States each year! This is in addition to the tons of nonaspirin pain relievers like acetaminophen (Tylenol) and other over-the-counter compounds that headache sufferers swallow every year.

Did you know that children get headaches, too—sometimes blinding and paralyzing headaches, and that slightly more males get migraine headaches as children, but more females get them as adults?

Are you aware that an estimated 300 medical conditions can cause headache? Some are serious, but fortunately most causes of headaches are not.

Did you know that headache is one of the most frequent reasons given by patients for visits to medical practitioners? It accounts for 10 million yearly office appointments with physicians (M.D. or D.O.) alone. This figure does not include visits to health care professionals who are not physicians, nor visits to chiropractors, hypnotists, acupuncturists, and other providers of nonmedical therapies.

You see, headache is a very real problem that affects millions of people!

Headache Has Always Been With Us

Headache is an ancient illness. Reference to it can be found in medical writings of Greek and Roman times. The ancient Greeks thought headaches were caused by demons and other evil spirits within the skull. The Romans believed that headaches and other painful discomforts were punishments inflicted by the gods. The Latin word *poena*, from which the word pain is derived, means penalty or punishment.

A variety of medieval therapies are found in historical documents. Among the more noteworthy was the application of rags soaked in vinegar and cow dung to the area of pain, the opening of the skull to release the evil spirits, the dripping of cocoa juice onto the painful area, and massaging the painful region with various animal parts including genitalia. Many of these strange-sounding practices have later proved to have a sound pharmocological basis. For example, the cocoa leaf has cocaine-like effects, and the genitals of beavers have been found to contain aspirin-like compounds.

How This Book Can Help You

This book reflects my awareness and respect for the immensity of the headache problem and the need to share currently available information with you. Among the things you will learn from this book are the basic causes of various headaches and the signs and symptoms of many headache disorders and problems related to them. I will explain the physical examination, medical history, and diagnostic tests that are needed to pinpoint or rule out any underlying disease or physical problem that could be causing your headache. In this book you will also find descriptions of acceptable treatments that are currently available for specific headache disorders.

I do not want you to treat your own headaches or to make diagnoses without the assistance of a skilled professional. The point is that the more you know, the better prepared you are to be a true partner with your doctor and other health care professionals. They cannot assume the entire task of taking care of you but must form an alliance with you based upon trust, communication, and persistence. Each individual with headache deserves to have his or her condition taken seriously and to be evaluated and treated with the same energy that is accorded other medical conditions. Even though the vast majority of headaches are not life threatening or destructive to the body, headache is a legitimate medical problem that can literally destroy the very quality and fiber of life.

The Situation Is More Hopeful Than Ever

During the past several years, the problem of headaches has received increasing attention. Specialty centers devoted to the treatment of this condition have sprung up throughout the country. In 1979, our outpatient center developed what was then the first hospital-based headache program in the world, devoted to those of our patients who simply could not obtain effective control without the intense and aggressive treatment that can be instituted in a hospital setting. Currently, we receive patients from all over the world who have spent years and sometimes fortunes seeking relief for their disabling headache condition. Recently, our hospital unit was awarded the first and only accreditation ever given to a center primarily devoted to the treatment of headache. We believe that this will initiate the establishment of standards for hospital programs devoted to the treatment of headaches.

For all of you with headache, there is new hope, there are new answers, new treatments, and new attitudes. Please do not assume that you must "live with it." Most of you can gain sufficient control over your headaches and other forms of head and neck pain so that they no longer compromise your ability to lead a normal life. Though the cause cannot always be stated with certainty, effective treatments can be found for most of you.

I hope that after reading this book you will have a better sense of the problem of headaches, and particularly a greater hope and enthusiasm for obtaining help and gaining control over this underestimated malady.

2

Kinds of Pain and Their Relationship to How the Brain Functions

When physicians describe medical conditions such as pain, they classify them in various ways. For example, a condition may be described as acute or chronic, primary or secondary.

Acute Versus Chronic Pain

Acute pain is relatively short-lived. It arises as a direct result of an identifiable cause and serves an alerting or protecting function. For example, a blow to the head may cause pain for a few minutes or several days. Acute pain generally diminishes spontaneously. Traditionally, pain has been approached and treated from the perspective of the acute pain model.

In contrast to acute pain, *chronic pain* is defined as pain that lasts or recurs over a period longer than six months. Usually, there is little or no identifiable disease or injury causing the painful symptoms. That is, acute pain is usually *secondary* to some other problem; chronic pain tends to be *primary*—a problem in itself. According to current thinking, chronic pain reflects a constellation of physiological and/or psychological disturbances that somehow alter the body's biological system for processing and coping with pain. Disturbances of this system result in continuing and/or recurring symptoms.

During the past ten years, scientific research has brought us better understanding of the biology of the brain. This increased knowledge has led to changing attitudes toward chronic pain. Emerging evidence suggests that chronic pain reflects an alteration in how the brain processes painful stimuli. Many authorities now believe that chronic pain occurs when a disturbance in the balance of various biological systems interacts with the emotional components of the mind. A person's vulnerability to this disruption may be acquired or inherited. Once activated, the pain cycle may be made worse by wide-ranging factors such as chronic stress, various other illnesses, trauma, or certain types of drugs. Chronic stress may also change the biological factors in the brain, making chronic pain more likely.

The Headache Syndrome

A syndrome is a combination of symptoms that occur together, combining to create an identifiable illness. Headache is defined as an uncomfortable sensation of the face, head, or neck area that is frequently described as throbbing, pressure-like, burning, stabbing, or searing. Like other pain syndromes, headache may be primary or secondary. Primary headaches (the chronic forms) include such familiar terms as migraine, so-called "tension" headache, and cluster headache, among others. These conditions reflect the presence of recurring or continuous headache symptoms that occur without an identifiable structural cause; that is, tests for organic disease are usually normal. The primary headache disorders occur with variable frequency and duration over a lifetime. Headaches may begin in early childhood or await onset until much later.

Secondary headaches are those that reflect an identifiable disease or abnormality. Thus, secondary headaches may signal the presence of a variety of conditions including infection and serious diseases of the spine or neck, including derangement of dental structures, brain tumors, aneurysms (blood vessel expansions), and others. Secondary headaches rarely produce continuing distress, because the pain is reduced once the underlying problem has been identified and treated.

Many persons experiencing recurring headaches have been led to believe that they have a principal cause for headache (such as sinus disease, neck arthritis, or jaw ailments). However, most people experiencing recurring headaches do not suffer from sufficient physical disease to account for the continuing and at times unrelenting pain. For example, some element of neck arthritis and/or jaw disturbance is common in people over 30, yet most of these individuals will not have headaches. Even if individuals do have minor changes in their necks or jaws, these changes are not necessarily the cause of their headaches, since common ailments may occur simultaneously.

Kinds of Headaches Discussed in This Book

In the past, the primary headaches were classified as specific syndromes on the basis of the presumed mechanism of pain. Now, recent medical reports and clinical observations have led many headache authorities to conclude that the clear and definite distinction between types of headaches may not be as firm as once believed. Many individuals with headache appear to pass through a spectrum of symptoms and headache forms during their lifetimes, moving from one headache syndrome to another or experiencing numerous headache types simultaneously. Nonetheless, for clarity and an appropriate perspective on treatment, the discussion in this book is arranged according to the traditional distinctions between headache syndromes. Among the headaches that we will review in this book are:

- Migraine
- Tension headache
- Cluster headache
- Daily chronic headache
- Posttraumatic headache
- Headaches in children
- Headaches resulting from disease

Who Gets Headaches and Why?

Although more is known about headaches than in the past, the cause of primary headaches is still not fully understood. Scientists had once presumed that migraine and cluster headache resulted from changes in blood vessel size—excessive dilation (expansion) and constriction. Tension headaches were presumed to occur from excessive contraction of head and neck muscles. However, it now appears that many, if not most, persons suffering from chronic and recurring headache are prone to them as a result of inherited tendencies. European researchers believe, particularly in the case of daily chronic headaches, that a progressive disturbance of certain brain chemical functions can be documented.

Although their theory is still unproven, many authorities propose that primary headaches result from a disturbance of brain chemistry or other physiological abnormalities that directly or indirectly affect the body's pain perception mechanism. In the presence of this tendency, head trauma, or acute and sustained emotional distress, some surgical procedures, physiological milestones such as childbirth and pregnancy, or the use of certain medicines such as oral contraceptives and antibiotics can activate headaches. A greater than expected likelihood of mood and sleep disturbances, and overuse of certain addicting substances, may also accompany this biological vulnerability. It is possible that the coexistence of these phenomena reflect disturbances of certain brain substances called neurotransmitters.

A Word About Brain Function

The brain is composed of nerve cells (neurons) and their extensions, together with supporting substance. All functions of the brain depend upon an interplay of certain brain chemicals, called *neurotransmitters*, which are secreted by the neurons. Current research suggests that certain diseases are caused by a deficiency or excess (inherited or acquired) of certain of these transmitters, or disturbance of their attachment sites called receptors. Among the illnesses now considered related to such disturbances are Parkinson's disease, Huntington's chorea, manic-depressive illness, inherited (biological) depression, certain types of epilepsy, some anxiety states, certain forms of dementia, and many others.

Since the 1950s, scientists have recognized that some forms of depression can be inherited and that they result from disturbances related to neurotransmitters. These substances are important in the control of mood and sleep function. In the middle 1970s, research showed that in addition to having its own "antidepressant transmitters" the brain also produced its own "painkiller," which had a remarkable similarity to morphine. Recognition that the brain produces such substances, called *endorphins*, represented a major breakthrough in recognizing how the brain's pain system might work. This mechanism also explained the important pain-controlling ability of morphine and narcotic-like substances. Recently, researchers tentatively demonstrated that the brain might also produce its own tranquilizers, which according to early data have a chemical structure similar to "Valium-like" tranquilizers. Researchers are currently considering whether certain yet unexplained disturbances of mood, neurological function, and other related problems including headache could reflect alterations of neurotransmitter function.

3

How Headache Problems Are Diagnosed

Over 300 medical conditions can cause headaches. Sometimes, a headache is a warning signal of serious disease, but statistics show that most recurring headaches are of the primary type (without serious implication). Even so, the physician must make sure that no illness that may produce headache is present. What kind of diagnostic evaluation you will receive depends on the health professional you choose.

Who Will Do the Testing?

Within the medical profession, a variety of specialists and generalists may be consulted to assess the cause of headaches. Each will use a diagnostic pathway consistent with the physician's own orientation and attitude about headaches. Most physicians, particularly specialists, have been trained to treat only those illnesses that are clearly identified by test results. In other words, they look for and treat acute secondary pain. Patients with primary headaches, after going through an elaborate series of evaluations, are often told that the tests are normal and that nothing can be found to account for their pain. Many patients report with disappointment and frustration that they are sent from specialist to specialist and yet despite hundreds and perhaps thousands of dollars in medical bills, nothing can be found and effective treatment has not been forthcoming.

This problem has many origins. First, the kinds of abnormalities associated with primary headaches are usually not identifiable with currently available testing procedures: Most recurring headaches are due to physiological, not structural, abnormalities. In addition, most physicians have been trained primarily to treat symptoms that can be documented on diagnostic testing. Moreover, the prevailing attitude toward headache and those who suffer from this illness discourages physicians from making a persistent effort at treating a subjective illness—that is, a problem that can be described but not clearly demonstrated. Patients with headaches are often presumed to be seeking tranquilizers or narcotics. There is also a widespread belief that patients with headache have emotional illness or excessive stress. These presumptions further compound the patient's problem.

Even though the traditional medical diagnostic systems have many shortcomings, I discourage seeking the assistance of nontraditional interventions or diagnostic evaluations until a thorough medical evaluation and treatment effort has been completed. The evaluations described below are the basic ones for headaches.

The Physical and History

A thorough history (data collection) and careful general and medical/neurological evaluation are necessary. General health background assessment can be critical to exclude a history of head injury, excessive medication usage, hormonal change, exposures to various toxins or substances, and much more. Specific features of headache and provoking and relieving factors can be important in the treatment program.

Special evaluations for ear, nasal, or throat conditions may be necessary, as are visual tests when eyes are suspected as a cause of discomfort. Similarly, a special evaluation of the teeth or jaw may be required in certain instances.

What is the psychological status of an individual? What about troubled family dynamics? With recurring headache, these factors cannot be overlooked. While the current trend is to view headaches as primarily a biological disturbance, psychiatric illness and stress-related problems can be important aggravating influences. Occasionally, they are a primary cause. An evaluation by a trained, experienced mental health professional is warranted in certain situations. However, it is no longer acceptable to presume that individuals experiencing recurring headaches possess psychological illness. Referring the patient to mental health professionals should take place only as a component of a comprehensive diagnostic and treatment plan.

Diagnostic Tests

Certain basic laboratory tests are virtually a routine part of headache evaluation. Others are recommended in specific instances.

Blood Tests Some of the diseases that can cause headache can be detected early in their course only by changes in blood chemistry and other components in the blood. I therefore recommend routine testing (screening) to consider obvious metabolic diseases. Among the conditions that must be considered are kidney and liver disease, diseases of the blood such as various anemias, disturbances of the endocrine system such as thyroid disease, and glucose abnormalities such as diabetes or hypoglycemia.

Radiologic Studies (X-rays) Routine x-rays of the head and neck demonstrate bony tissue and are only minimally helpful in identifying most of the important causes of headache. More advanced techniques have largely replaced simple x-rays, although these techniques do tend to be more expensive. Except for certain conditions, the simple skull x-ray is of minimal value compared with the CT scan (see below). X-rays of the neck can show significant disturbances of vertebral structures, but the neck is not the primary cause of headache in most individuals. The neck x-ray should be used selectively. Sinus x-rays can demonstrate infection in the sinuses, but these studies should be reserved for patients who have other symptoms suggesting sinus infection.

Electroencephalography (EEG) Headache authorities are divided in opinion on the value of EEG and related neuroelectrical studies. The EEG can show certain disturbances of brain function, irregularities of rhythm, the presence of seizure-like activity, and the effects of drugs or other metabolic disturbances on the nervous system. Some authorities use the EEG, which is much less expensive than a CT scan, to screen for the need to do a CT scan.

Spinal Taps Spinal taps are generally not necessary in most patients who have recurring headache. They should be done only when serious concern for the presence of infection or bleeding within the central nervous system exists.

Computed Axial Tomography (CT Scan, CAT Scan) The CT scan, sometimes called a CAT scan, represents the most effective way to assess for an intracranial (inside the head) condition that causes headache. This technique consists of computerized x-ray evaluation that radiographically "slices" the brain into various parts, allowing for evaluation of many brain structures heretofore not detectable by routine evaluation. The risks of CT scanning are not great. X-ray exposure is generally only slightly more than with a routine skull x-ray. To improve the efficiency of interpretation, an intravenous injection of contrast material is frequently advised. A patient with a history of allergy to shellfish or to contrast material will either be pretreated to avoid allergic reaction or will not undergo this component of the test.

The CT scan can identify most but not all structural intracranial causes of headache. It does not generally identify aneurysm (blood vessel ballooning), however. Most authorities agree that the CT scan offers a major advance in the ability to detect causes of headache. Only the more recently developed magnetic resonance imaging (MRI) or positron emission tomography (PET scanning) are more advanced techniques, but these are not appropriate for routine use.

The Pros and Cons of CT Scanning

While few would argue against using the CT scan in specific circumstances, it is less clear whether all patients with recurring headaches should undergo a CT scan evaluation. Proponents assert that CT scans will identify abnormalities that cannot be detected in any other way and that they will reveal disturbances that could be life threatening if not identified and treated early. Moreover, proponents argue that until the CT scan is done, attempts to control pain are inappropriate and complacency that recurring headache is not serious is inappropriate. They cite numerous case examples to support this concern. In addition, patient anxiety and uncertainty resulting from the failure of early treatments to bring about relief, and the frequent but often unspoken fear that a brain tumor or serious disease is present, subjects the patient to unnecessary stress that may actually make the headaches worse.

Those who believe that CT scans should not be used for most cases of recurring headache argue that the CT scan is an expensive procedure (between $250 and $450). They also assert that it should be done only when specific indications for the test are present. They point out that most individuals undergoing CT scans have normal results, and therefore relatively few CT scans are of actual value in determining treatment course.

The issue is further complicated by some insurance companies who refuse to pay for CT scans except when the physician certifies the likely presence of a serious disease, which generally cannot be established *until* the CT scan is done. In several states, patients who have undergone CT scans on the advice of their physicians have received letters from the insurance companies stating that the CT scan will not be paid for because headaches are not sufficient justification for this test. These letters suggest either obliquely or directly that the physicians were excessive in their testing procedures.

Physicians argue that they are caught in the middle. They

are held by medical, legal, and ethical standards to make certain that all causes are considered. They have been legally held accountable when CT scans were delayed until specific criteria were met, later showing the presence of a disease that could have been diagnosed earlier had the test been done sooner. Between patient care concerns and medical/legal considerations on the one hand and insurance companies and cost containment pressures on another, physicians are divided in their opinion on CT scans. Thus, inconsistency and disagreement about the appropriate criteria for the CT scan in the pursuit of headache symptoms is common.

It is my opinion that most patients with frequent or complicated headaches require a CT scan. Failure to do this test early in the course of illness does present a risk, however slight, of a serious or even fatal delay in establishing proper diagnosis. While it is acknowledged that most patients with headache will have normal test results, numerous case examples can be cited in which the opposite is true and in which delay could have or did result in serious outcomes. Certainty that a serious disease is absent cannot be established without a CT scan. Moreover, I believe that because many health care dollars can be saved by early and effective evaluation and treatment of headaches, the additional expense for a CT scan is worthwhile and is compensated for by the savings. The risks of such a test are minimal.

4

Understanding the Basic Features of Migraine Headache

Migraine is the most widely studied of all headache types, yet it is also the most widely misunderstood. Both health professionals and the public are plagued by myths about this illness, which was recognized as early as the second century A.D. Aretaeus of Cappadocia (second century A.D.) is credited with the initial recognition of a headache syndrome affecting one side of the head and often accompanied by gastrointestinal distress and visual disturbances. The Greeks called in *hemikranios* (half head), which became the *hemicranium* in Latin, "megrim," in Old English, and migraine in French and in modern U.S. usage. Patients may describe it as "blinding headache," "sick headache," or

"migrant headache." ⌐Despite its long history, the precise
mechanism that causes migraine continues to elude researchers.

Some Facts and Features

Prevalence Attempts to determine accurate epidemiological data for migraine are frustrated by the absence of universally agreed upon diagnostic criteria. Despite several attempts to establish consistent criteria for the diagnosis of migraine, general agreement does not currently exist.

In 1962, one researcher reported on studies of 9000 Swedish children and demonstrated a prevalence of migraine ranging from 1% by six years of age to 5% at 15 years of age. In 1970, other researchers studying several thousand Danish children suggested that by age 40, 19% of women experienced migraine. It has been suggested that as many as 15% to 19% of men and 25% to 29% of women may experience a migraine attack during their lifetime. Two researchers estimate that eight to 12 million Americans suffer from migraine. Migraine does not consistently vary with respect to race, education, or social class.

Male:Female Distribution About 75% of migraine sufferers are women, the highest number of cases occurring during hormonally active, reproductive years. The female to male ratio of migraine is estimated at 3 to 1 in adult life. For children, the male:female ratio is more equal. Perhaps males with migraine may more likely experience an end of their attacks before adulthood. It is also possible that more females than males experience their first attack after childhood (see Chapter 12).

In one study, which demonstrated a 5% prevalence by age 15, notable differences were demonstrated between boys and girls with respect to degree of disability and impairment of daily living. The data suggested that school time lost by boys with migraine did not differ substantially from that of boys without migraine. Girls with migraine lose much more time from school than females not reporting headache.

Age of Onset and Course Migraine may first develop at any time during life. However, the second and third decades (ages 10 through 30) are most often cited. Peak ages are 21 to 30, 41 to 45, and 51 to 55. Migraine can occur in children as young or younger than three years of age! One-quarter to one-third of patients with migraine experience their first symptoms before 10 years of age. By age 30, approximately 75% of people who get migraine headaches have experienced their first attack. Occasionally, the first migraine occurs after age 50. Migraine in remission for many years may reappear after decades of quiescence.

Migraine is an intermittent illness, and its natural history is distinguished by its variability. A strong tendency for pattern change exists throughout life in terms of frequency, symptom development, and sensitivity to provoking factors. In a follow-up of one original study, 60% of adult patients with childhood migraine were still having migraine attacks. The attacks seemed less intense and less frequent.

In early childhood, migraine may not possess typical adult features but may be characterized instead by *migraine equivalents*. These are nonheadache symptoms which reflect the blood vessel and body organ excitability in migraine-prone patients that are discussed in Chapter 11. During later years of life, migraine equivalents rather than typical headache attacks may once again prevail.

Patients exhibiting typical migraine attacks early in life may experience muscle contraction–like headaches later on (see Chapters 9 and 10), reflecting perhaps a shift from blood-vessel mechanisms moderated by the autonomic nervous system to muscular or central nervous system mechanisms. Two researchers were unable to demonstrate a decrease of headache frequency or intensity after menopause. Women taking hormones (estrogens) after menopause may be more likely to experience intense episodic migraine.

Hereditary Factors

Ninety percent of migraine patients report a parent, aunt or uncle, or grandparent with migraine. Additionally, patients report family members with sick headaches, sinus headaches, tension headaches, and blinding headaches, some of which are likely to represent migraine. Most patients report migraine on the mother's side.

Classification and Definition

In 1962, a group of researchers, attempting to encourage uniformity in the diganosis of chronic headache, proposed guidelines for the diagnosis of migraine and other headache disorders. Despite this energetic effort and those of others, the diagnosis of migraine continues to be established arbitrarily and inconsistently by researchers and clinicians alike.

Migraine is an inherited periodic disorder characterized by recurring attacks of wide-ranging symptoms, most notably headache. The headache varies in intensity, associated symptoms, frequency, and duration. Gastrointestinal distress and visual disturbances, though not necessarily present, are the most common associated problems.

Migraine has historically been divided into two distinct subtypes, *classic* and *common*. The distinction between these two entities on biological grounds is not clear. Some authors prefer to explain both classic and common migraine as related biological events, occurring along a continuum of biological expression, while others maintain that classic and common migraine are distinct and separate illnesses.

Classic Migraine Classic migraine is a two-phase disorder in which an aura (preheadache period) characterized by temporary neurological phenomena lasting 15 to 30 minutes is followed by unilateral or bilateral headache. Although the neurological symptoms usually occur before the headache, they may develop during the headache or following its termination. Classic migraine accounts for 15 to 20% of migraine attacks.

Classic migraine can be further defined according to symptoms and where it strikes. For instance, one form is paralytic, one form impairs the ability to express language (aphasic migraine), another form causes double vision and paralysis of eye movement, and still another form impairs sensation, causing numbness. Many other forms of migraine also exist including a form that causes loss of consciousness and one that causes imbalance and dizziness. Loss of equilibrium, disturbances of balance, double vision, and even coma can occur in a form of migraine referred to as *vertebrobasilar* migraine. This name reflects the presumed location of symptom origin, the brain stem.

The visual disturbances associated with classic migraine (blindness, flashing dots and patterns, and others) are thought to be caused by impairment of the back portion of the brain, the occipital lobe.

The term *complicated migraine* refers variably to either persisting neurological symptoms that remain after the termination of the headache or to extremely intense, dramatic neurological impairment, occurring during the headache or preceding it. Many times, "complicated migraine" mimics an actual stroke, and it is sometimes misdiagnosed as such.

Common Migraine Common migraine (nonclassic migraine) is not associated with well-defined focal neurological disturbances during or preceding the headache. However, those with recurring common migraine may experience various vague, nondistinct emotional, gastrointestinal, and organ disturbances before or during the headache.

Signs and Symptoms of Migraine

Migraine is most often accompanied by pain. Some attacks occur without headache and the headache may also exist alone. More commonly, it is accompanied by gastrointestinal distress (nausea and vomiting), visual and sensory disturbances, and events such as depression, malaise, and fatigue.

How the Headache Manifests Itself

Quality of the Pain Most, but not all migraine attacks are accompanied by headache. The headache is one-sided (unilateral) in over two-thirds of the attacks and on both sides (bilateral) in the remainder. In its earliest stages, the pain is irritational and dull, soon evolving into a throbbing discomfort. As it intensifies and persists, a boring, aching, nonthrobbing discomfort prevails. Lifting, bending, or straining usually intensifies the discomfort.

Pain intensity can vary from attack to attack, and fluctuation during the attack is common. A migraine may be mild and annoying or distinctively incapacitating. Occasionally, sharp "ice pick" jabs occur around the eye socket or temple. This sudden attack may occur at times other than during a typical headache in over a third of migraine patients.

Location of the Pain The pain is frequently located in an eye, temple, or frontal region. It may remain localized or may radiate over half or all of the head, frequently enlisting muscle aching from the neck and shoulders. Many report the onset of headache in the neck and shoulders with radiation to the forehead. Facial attacks (facial migraine) with similarity to other migraine episodes except for the facial location can occur.

Most people experiencing unilateral pain during an attack will have an alteration of sidedness on at least some occasions. The pain may recur consistently on the same side in approximately 20% of patients.

Other Characteristics of the Attack The headache may begin at any time, day or night. Awakening during the night because of a headache is common, as is waking early in the morning with an evolving attack. Because the preheadache aura of classic migraine rarely awakens its victim and cannot be felt during sleep, it is difficult to assess the frequency of classic migraine during sleep. Reports that a mood disturbance, appetite change with specific food craving, and changes in thirst occurring the evening before the attack are common.

Those experiencing the mixed headache syndrome (see Chapter 10) may report that a severe headache (migraine) occurs whenever the daily ingestion of analgesics (painkilling drugs) is reduced, an argument used to justify their continued preventive use of analgesics in a "preventive" mode.

Most people experiencing migraine will encounter between one and four attacks per month, although variability and even "clustering" is common. Migraine does not typically occur daily, every other day, or even several times during a week. Those experiencing more than one or two separate attacks per week are ususaly found to be overusing ergot medication and "rebounding," consuming another migraine-provoking substance, experiencing hormonal disturbances, or undergoing intense emotional duress.

Migraine may crescendo and descrescendo prior to subsiding, but it generally lasts for less than one day in approximately two-thirds of its victims. Nevertheless, three-to four-day attacks are not uncommon. Following an attack, lethargy and fatigue may persist for a day or longer.

Pain other than headache may occur during a migraine attack or may develop between attacks. Chest pain, abdominal distress, and pain in the extremities are common.

Common Symptoms That Accompany Migraine Headache

Although headache is typically the most dramatic event in migraine, it is one of several distressing symptoms. Scalp tenderness, general weakness or discomfort, lightheadedness, and dizziness occur in many people. Depression, inappropriate lassitude or hyperactivity, mental cloudiness, irritability, exhilaration, and food craving—particularly for sweets and chocolate—may precede, accompany, or follow both the classic and the common migraine attacks and may actually herald migraine by as much as a day or longer (see below).

Visual disturbances of a greater or lesser degree are the most common associated problems accompanying a migraine. Approximately 80% of people with migraine experience heightened and often disagreeable sensitivity to light during an attack. Blurred vision is common, as are "shimmering" or "floating" visual images.

In addition to visual disturbances, gastrointestinal distress occurs frequently. Nausea and vomiting are present in over one half of patients during an attack, and diarrhea in approximately 20%. Anorexia (lack of appetite), abdominal cramping, or simply a queasy feeling is often present. The nausea and vomiting originate in the brain centers, not the stomach, and the diarrhea may be related to the effects of the neurotransmitter serotonin on the gastrointestinal tract. Loss of consciousness, dizziness, and disorientation occur in migraine, as can acute confusional states which may precede the migraine episodes.

Other generalized alterations in migraine include changes in blood pressure and pulse rate, pallor of the skin with localized or generalized edema (swelling), blood vessel narrowing (vasoconstriction), chills, fever, nasal stuffiness, changes in the eye pupils, and lacrimation (tearing). Facial temperature during an attack may be cooler on the affected side. Nosebleeds and bleeding in or around an eye are possible.

Migraine Equivalents

Migraine equivalents (see Chapter 11) are nonheadache, periodic disturbances in individuals predisposed to having migraines. Among the migraine equivalents are vertigo (spinning imbalance), gastrointestinal distress, a tendency toward motion sickness, periodic fainting, flashing or flickering of lights, tachycardia (rapid heartbeat), mood disturbances, and other body and nerve sensations. A clue to the diagnosis of migraine equivalents is that they are likely to be precipitated by events known to provoke migraine.

One researcher has drawn attention to the presence of nonneurological symptoms resulting from migraine but not involving headache that begin after middle age. These short-lived neurological symptoms tend to resemble stroke-like symptoms called transient ischemic attacks (TIAs). This researcher employed the term *transient migraine accompaniments* (TMAs) to identify these neurological disturbances and distinguish them from those occurring as a consequence of stroke-like illness. This subject is discussed later in this book.

Specific Nervous System Disturbances in Migraine

Neurological (nervous-system) disturbances are commonly encountered in migraine. They can affect the muscles, sensation, vision, and other brain functions. Generally, these disturbances occur as part of the aura, the heralding events of classic migraine, although they may occur with the headache and sometimes after the headache. These disturbances, when occurring as part of the aura, generally last only 15 to 30 minutes and are seen in approximately 15 to 20% of people with migraine.

Historically, these neurological disturbances were thought to be due to a reduction of blood circulation. Recently, some researchers have suggested that the reduction in blood flow itself may be a consequence of a primary abnormality of brain function. This abnormality, periodic and not progressive, may be inherited.

Visual Disturbances Virtually no part of the brain is spared involvement in migraine, but certain areas appear more vulnerable. The most common neurological symptom in migraine involves the visual system. Flashing lights, visual hallucinations, blind spots, and other disturbances are reported. The *fortification spectrum* represents a pattern of glittering zigzag lines and points that many migraine sufferers experience. This zigzag pattern resembles the fortification barriers constructed around embattled cities in older times, hence its name. Though one senses the disturbance in the eyes, the actual abnormality arises somewhere in the brain. Ironically, these visual disturbances have been reported in patients who have been totally blind and in one woman with both eyes removed.

The *Alice-in-Wonderland phenomenon* refers to the bizarre alterations in shape, color, size, and body image that may occur during some migraine attacks. In addition to visual disturbances, alterations in smell and taste may be present. Approximately one-fourth of patients with migraine will report flashes of color and noncolor images. The suggestion that the bizarre disturbances of this syndrome reflect personal experiences of Lewis J. Carroll, the author of *Alice in Wonderland* and a migraine victim, has considerable appeal. However, one researcher suggests that Alice's adventures in Wonderland may have been written before Lewis Carroll experienced his first migraine.

Attacks of weakness on one side or both sides together with symptoms of numbness and sensory loss can also accompany or occur in advance of a migraine attack. Moreover, some patients with migraine have difficulty speaking. Some experience changes in their mood—anger, depression, or even exhilaration—before, during, or after a migraine attack. Seizures may also occur during migraine.

Finally, a researcher in England has suggested that migraine may actually begin many days before the headache occurs. Many of his patients repeatedly experienced mood change, including periods of depression or anger, occurring several days before the headache is first noticed. In addition, following a severe headache individuals may experience a day of lethargy or fatigue. Most physicians now recognize migraine may indeed span three, four, or even five days of time and that many symptoms, otherwise not easily classified, may occur in advance of the ensuing headache.

In summary, patients with migraine may experience a wide array of neurological deficits, many times mimicking a stroke. The disturbances may be mental (depression, mood swings, anger, exhilaration) or may reflect paralysis or sensory disturbances. Imbalance, double vision, loss of consciousness, seizures, confusion, inability to speak, and many others are possible. One childhood form of migraine actually causes confusion lasting many hours along with increased sedation and at times stupor. Many of these children have been thought to have emotional problems, and only later was it discovered that they were affected by a periodic form of migraine.

Neurological disturbances in migraine are generally short-lived, but occasionally they become permanent and actually result in a stroke. This seems to occur quite infrequently, given the large number of patients who experience migraine. Nonetheless, patients with migraines accompanied by neurological symptoms are strongly advised to stop smoking, to reduce their consumption of fats if their blood levels of cholesterol and triglycerides are high, and to avoid the use of birth control pills or other types of hormones unless absolutely necessary, since these factors appear to enhance the risk of stroke.

Making the Diagnosis of Migraine

Many disorders can produce migraine-like symptoms, just as migraine might mimic other conditions. Your doctor must consider a wide array of important and sometimes serious diseases before the diagnosis of migraine can be established with certainty. Among these are stroke-related illnesses, hypoglycemia, certain disturbances of various body organs, aneurysms (ballooned blood vessels), epilepsy, congenital malformations of arteries and veins, tumors, lupus erythematosis, glaucoma, and certain forms of heart disease.

5

Factors That Trigger Migraine Headache

This chapter is devoted to a review of those influences that medical researchers believe precipitate (trigger) individual migraine attacks. Much more than is currently known must be learned about the origin and development of migraine and the many influences upon an attack before a complete explanation is possible. Nevertheless, recognition that certain influences are capable of provoking a migraine attack aids in establishing a diagnosis and in planning a treatment program. Certain precipitating influences such as a menstrual period, ingestion of alcohol, or sleeping later than usual are so characteristic in their ability to provoke a migraine that establishing that they were present prior to the onset of a headache may clearly identify the headache as migraine.

The evolution of a migraine attack is a complex process involving many factors. Isolating and controlling these provoking influences, when possible, does not necessarily bring about the prevention of headaches, but some patients, by eliminating and avoiding some of these influences, appear to experience an overall improvement in the course of their attacks. For example, discontinuing birth control pills when headaches appear aggravated by them, awakening no later on the weekends than during the week, and avoiding alcohol when sensitive to it may well provide dramatic benefit to some individuals.

Complicating an accurate evaluation of precipitating factors is that most people with migraine experience a changing susceptibility to these and other stimuli, so that the provoking events may exert an inconsistent and variable influence during migraine years. This variability may be related to changing internal physiological events. One researcher, studying several thousand patients with migraine, demonstrated that vulnerability to food substances seemed much greater during premenstrual and menstrual days than during other times of the cycle.

The variability and inconsistency of precipitating factors makes it difficult to isolate with any degree of reliability the many biological and nonbiological influences on migraine. Most specialists agree, however, that careful attention to these influences is justifiable in the care of migraine patients and the understanding of this disorder.

The prevailing attitude on migraine origin and development (see Chapter 6) is that migraine represents the clinical consequence of a biological predisposition combined with exaggerated reactivity—rendering the migraine patient more vulnerable to many external as well as internal influences. This vulnerability appears to fluctuate periodically or perhaps in cycles, greatly influencing the individual's susceptibility to precipitating events.

The following discussion will review many of the precipitating influences on migraine (Table 1). Most common among these are emotional factors, hormonal changes in women, dietary influences, sleep, and glandular and chemical changes. It must be emphasized that these influences may have no effect on a particular person with migraine, may have a partial effect requiring the presence of more than one circumstance or influence in order for an attack to ensue, or may alone be able to provoke an attack. It is most likely that several factors must be simultaneously present, having a cumulative influence on the biological circumstances responsible for migraine.

TABLE 1

Some Possible Migraine-Provoking Influences

Psychological
  stress/anxiety
  anger
  "letdown"
  exhilaration
	Sleep
	  too much
	  too little
	  napping

Dazzling light	Dietary*

Hormonal
  menarche
  menstruation
  menopause
  pregnancy (first trimester)
  delivery
  birth control pills
  externally administered
    estrogens
	Certain medicines
	
	Marked weather changes
	
	Head/Neck trauma
	  mild
	  severe
	
	Toxins

*See Table 2

Psychological and Emotional Factors

Emotional dynamics play an important role in triggering many migraine attacks. Prolonged stress, internalized hostilities, and a wide variety of other emotional and personality factors appear important in many but not all migraine patients.

Physicians have traditionally focused on the so-called "migraine personality," which is supposed to be characterized by compulsive, perfectionistic, rigid, and achievement-driven elements, often accompanied by internalized anger and excessive self-control. This emphasis may not be warranted. Many migraine patients indeed have obsessive, compulsive, and aggressive personality features, often accompanied by an inability to express hostile feelings openly. However, many others do not possess these characteristics. Moreover, many individuals without migraine have "migraine personalities"—the hard-driving personality commonly called Type A.

In a study of 100 persons experiencing migraine, over one-half suffered their first migraine during a period of emotional stress. However, this study, like others, was unable to find convincing evidence that migraine sufferers were more neurotic than other people. Persons suffering migraine may, by virtue of several factors, be predisposed to excessive reactions to stressful events.

Intense stress, particularly that associated with rage and resentment for which full expression is lacking and which may accumulate, can trigger an attack. The person who gets migraine headaches may be biologically more likely to respond to these factors in such a way as to induce a headache. Individuals with compulsive personality traits and the often accompanying ambitious, perfectionistic, and orderly features may possess a stressful bias to their personality, which in the appropriate biological setting gives way to migraine events.

While stress is important, just as many people, perhaps even more, may experience migraine in a period of "letdown" *after* the stress has subsided. Many will state that headaches occur after the stress is terminated—for example, on the first day of a vacation (holiday headache) or on the weekend after an intense week and sustained emotional duress.

A discussion of the biochemistry of depression and stress is well beyond the scope of this chapter. However, it is appropriate to mention that a biological relationship among depression, stress, and chronic pain may exist. There may be a greater than expected association of headache and depression.

In summary, stress, depression, anxiety, and anger as well as "letdown" after intense emotional events can all provoke headache attacks. Although the biological aspects of these adverse psychological states are not well understood, there is little doubt that intense emotions, perhaps via both central (brain) and peripheral mechanisms, exert an influence on headache provocation.

Hormonal Factors

Migraine in women usually worsens during times of hormonal change, such as menarche (the onset of the menstrual cycle at puberty), menstruation, ovulation, and menopause.

Menstruation Up to 60% of female migraine sufferers report migraine attacks just before, during, or after their menstrual periods. Approximately 14% experience headache exclusively around the time of menstruation. Many of these women may be more likely to have had their first migraine attack in their early teens at the time of menarche, and to experience improvement of their migraine during pregnancy.

Our understanding of *menstrual migraine* has been aided by the work of Dr. B. W. Somerville, who identified the reduction of plasma estrogen as one important factor influencing the precipitation of a menstrual migraine. He demonstrated that the menstrual headache could be delayed by the administration of estrogen but not by the administration of progesterone.

Many women will experience the first migraine attack at or around their first menstrual period. In some, the initial migraine event is characterized by a prolonged vascular headache attack, unresponsive to medicine appropriate for migraine, and which after several weeks terminates spontaneously. This prolonged attack gives way to more typical periodic migraine events.

Pregnancy Pregnancy has a variable effect on migraine. Although existing migraine often intensifies during the first trimester, over 70% of women will experience an improvement during the second and third trimester. Following delivery, however, headache may return within hours to days. A woman's very first migraine attack may also occur shortly after delivery. Migraine in remission since childhood or adolescence may return during pregnancy, particularly the first. In one recent study, 15 out of 40 women on a postnatal ward experienced headaches in the first postpartum week, usually between the third and sixth days. Among women with a previous history of migraine the rate of these headaches was higher. Rapidly falling estrogen and progesterone levels, or alterations in serotonin metabolism were suggested as possible factors.

One researcher, emphasizing the "euphoria" experienced

by many women in the third trimester, suggests that headache improvement as well as the heightened emotions of pregnancy may be due to the increased activity of the morphine-like brain chemicals called endorphins that occurs in pregnancy.

Birth Control Pills In general, birth control pills will increase the frequency and severity of migraine attacks. Many women not experiencing migraine previously will experience their first attack soon after starting birth control pills. It is estimated that at least half of those experiencing headaches while taking birth control pills did not experience headaches prior to their use. Many women report that headache was the primary motivation for discontinuing the pill. A minority experience an improvement in headache frequency while taking birth control pills.

Most women experiencing an intensification or precipitation of their headaches from birth control pills do so in the earlier states of use, usually within the first several months. In those experiencing a worsening of attacks, discontinuance of the "pill" brings about improvement in up to 70%. The improvement occurs over months and is not generally immediate.

Migraine may be associated with an increased risk of stroke. Oral contraceptives and estrogen also enhance stroke risk. Women with migraine taking oral contraceptives and other estrogen preparations and who also smoke cigarettes may have a substantially increased risk of developing stroke and other disorders related to obstruction of the blood vessels.

Menopause The influence of menopause on migraine is variable. Migraine may disappear at the time of menopause in some women. An intensification of vascular headaches may occur in others. Many women with distinct episodic vascular headaches in earlier years will experience the evolution to a more daily muscular-like headache process just prior to, during, or after menopause. This headache may become the dominant pain pattern during later years of life (see Chapters 9 and 10).

Hysterectomy and Headache Hysterectomy does not generally lessen migraine. Furthermore, the use of estrogens, even when the ovaries are removed, may aggravate preexisting migraine.

Women with headaches who must employ estrogen after menopause may benefit from the use of synthetic preparations instead of conjugated forms derived from animal sources. Low-dose therapy is recommended. Although estrogen replacement generally aggravates vascular headache tendencies, some women improve with estrogen administration.

The evidence seems to suggest that women predisposed to migraine are likely to experience an increase in migraine frequency and intensity during times of either estrogen elevation or decrease. Most notable is the reduction of estrogen at menstruation, the enhancement associated with oral contraceptive use, that during the first trimester of pregnancy, and the increase when estrogens are administered as drugs.

The risk of stroke in women with migraine who also use oral contraceptives may be greater than that associated with chance alone. Women suffering migraine should be advised to avoid oral contraceptives. This is particularly important in those women who smoke and in whom the use of estrogen-containing preparations is accompanied by an increase in migraine frequency or intensity.

Sleep

People with migraine, like those suffering from other vascular headaches, may be awakened from sleep by a headache. Nighttime sleep and daytime napping are well recognized precipitants to migraine. Many people will cite either too much or too little sleep as a provoking influence for their headaches.

Among the various stages of sleep, rapid eye movement (REM) sleep (dream sleep) has been most associated with headache arousal. Rapid eye movement sleep is that phase accompanied by rapid eye movements, in conjunction with lower voltage, high frequency electroencephalographic (EEG) patterns, and a variety of physiological events including elevated heart rate, increased blood flow to the brain, rapid respiration, and dreaming. In adults, REM sleep accounts for approximately 25% of sleeping time, whereas in infancy and childhood REM sleep may dominate sleeping hours.

Patients with migraine frequently report that awakening one or two hours later than usual will often be associated with headache. For this reason, people with migraine are best advised to awaken at the same time each day. Awakening early, eating a small breakfast, and then returning to bed may be acceptable for some.

In summary, sleep may provoke migraine, and this may be related to the nature and extent of the various stages of sleep, the metabolic changes that occur, cerebral blood flow patterns, increased brain metabolism, alterations in respiration, oxygenation, and glucose levels, and fluctuations in serotonin and other brain chemicals during sleep. Similarly, the influence of intense emotional experiences during dream states must be considered.

Dietary Influences on Migraine

The relationship of eating habits and certain foods to migraine precipitation is not well understood. Neither is there general agreement on existing data. Approximately 25% of surveyed individuals associate a food with headache onset.

Fasting and Altered Blood Sugar Metabolism Fasting or missing meals is an important aggravating influence for headache in some individuals. In a study of over 2000 women with migraine, the absence of food for five or more hours during wakefulness or 13 overnight had been present in the majority of those in whom a migraine attack subsequently developed. This study also demonstrated an enhanced vulnerability to presumed dietary aggravating substances (see below) during a menstrual period.

The mechanism by which fasting provokes a headache remains uncertain. Hypoglycemia ("low blood sugar"), when present, can result in vasodilatation (widening of the vessels, in particular, the arteries), and a vascular headache is a presumed consequence. Fasting, even in the absence of hypoglycemia, affects brain serotonin turnover and other physiological reactions.

Fasting and altered glucose metabolism may be influential in precipitating a migraine attack and lowering the threshold to other aggravating factors. Those who suffer from migraines—with and without abnormalities of glucose metabolism—should be advised to eat regularly and to avoid simple carbohydrates (sugars). (See Chapter 14 for further discussion of hypoglycemia.)

Tyramine and Related Amines Since the early 1900s, tyramine and other dietary amines have been linked to the precipitation of headaches. (Amines are a group of compounds derived from ammonia.) Table 2 lists many of the foods containing one or more of these substances. Amines may influence the release of serotonin from blood platelets. They are also thought to affect the expansion and constriction of the blood vessels.

The actual importance of amines in triggering migraine is of considerable controversy. Studies demonstrating a relation-

TABLE 2

Some Possible Food Triggers

Foods containing tyramine
  chocolate
  aged cheese
  vinegar
    relishes
    dressings
    sauces
    catsup
  liver, kidney, organs
  alcohol (see below)
  sour cream
  yogurt
  yeast extracts
  others
	Alcohol products
	  wine/champagne
	  liquor, beer
	
	Fatty foods
	
	Foods containing nitrite
	  (a preservative)
	  hot dogs
	  sandwich meats
	  others

Citrus fruits
 	
Milk and milk products
	Foods containing monosodium
	  glutamate (MSG)
	
	Caffeine
	  too much
	  "rebound"

Onions	Seafood Nutrasweet artificial sweetener (contains phenylalanine)

ship between the ingestion of these chemicals and the precipitation of migraine have been seriously challenged by others questioning the reliability of this effect.

This issue remains unsettled. Some patients who associate the onset of headache with the ingestion of certain types of foods report that prior to the onset of an attack there will be a distinct craving for certain types of foods, particularly chocolate and other sweets.

It is possible that the craving itself is caused by the changes that have begun in the brain, particularly those that affect the appetite center (the hypothalamus). Thus, disturbances in the brain cause changes in appetite (cravings) that some people have misinterpreted as causing the headache that is really a result of changes in the brain.

Alcohol Alcohol is a nonspecific expander of blood vessels, and this effect probably accounts for its headache-provoking capacity. Liquor also contains varying amounts of tyramine and frequently histamine. Blood-vessel dilation is presumed to result from alcohol's influence on the central nervous system (brain and spinal cord). Alcohol is one of the few dietary factors reliably demonstrated to trigger migraine.

In people with migraine, the least likely headache-provoking beverages seem to be blended whiskeys, Scotch, vodka, and Sauterne and Riesling wines. Red wine and brandy are likely to be the most provoking (see Chapter 15 for an additional discussion on alcohol). Recently, researchers have discovered that some drugs similar to those used to treat arthritis, when taken before ingestion of alcohol, can sometimes prevent the development of alcohol-related pain, including some of the elements of the hangover (see Chapter 7).

Nitrites Nitrites and related compounds, employed in many food items to create a pink color and impart a cured flavor, have blood-vessel dilating actions that can provoke migraine-like headaches in some persons. These additives are found in such commonly eaten items as smoked fish, bologna, pepperoni, bacon, frankfurters, corned beef, pastrami, canned ham, and sausages. It is estimated that 12 billion pounds of nitrite are currently added to food in the United States yearly. This chemical was used in early Roman days in brine to cure meat and in early Asia as a food preservative and dessert component.

The nitrite-induced headache is usually felt in both temples. It is dull and throbbing, and it generally occurs within 30 minutes after ingestion. Although similar to migraine, it is uncertain whether this attack actually represents a migrainous event or is a nonspecific vascular headache occurring in people predisposed to migraine.

Monosodium Glutamate Monosodium glutamate (MSG) is a natural component of protein that is suspected of being a neurotransmitter, and precursor to gamma aminobutyric acid (GABA). It may release acetylcholine, a chemical that stimulates muscle function, and it is capable of inhibiting absorption of glucose (blood sugar) by brain cells. An estimated 20,000 tons of MSG are added to food yearly. It is sold in food stores under the trade name Accent and is used in such commonly ingested items as Chinese food, processed foods, dry roasted nuts, soups, sauces, and potato chip products.

In the late 1960s Dr. H. H. Schaumberg, a Chinese food enthusiast, identified monosodium glutamate as the provoking agent for what came to be called *Chinese restaurant syndrome*. This syndrome includes the symptoms of substernal pressure and burning sensations; pain about the head, neck, and eyes; flushing; sweating; and mood disturbances. In sensitive individuals, these symptoms occur within 15 to 25 minutes after the ingestion of MSG.

The number of people actually sensitive to MSG is unknown. Avoidance of MSG appears to prevent headaches without the aid of any medication in several patients I have personally encountered. In each, the headaches were intense and throbbing, located bilaterally or unilaterally, and occurred within 15 to 20 minutes following the ingestion of dietary MSG. It is possible that persons vulnerable to MSG reactions do not metabolize (digest) it properly.

Caffeine Caffeine induces many adverse physiological responses, and the syndrome of caffeinism is well documented. Caffeinism may be insidious, and individual susceptibility varies. Caffeine peaks in the blood 30 to 45 minutes after oral ingestion and its effects can last for two and one-half hours or longer. A variety of symptoms including mood disturbances with anxiety-related symptomatology, sleep disturbances, and headache can result from excessive use of caffeine and withdrawal from it.

The headache caused by excessive use of caffeine or withdrawal from it is usually a throbbing, which in the case of withdrawal occurs between 12 and 24 hours after the last ingestion. The headaches are in some ways similar to migraine pain. They cannot accurately be called migraine but may be more likely to occur in individuals predisposed to migraine. (See Chapter 18 for more on caffeine.)

Other Foods Other foods may precipitate migraine-like headaches. Among the most commonly identified substances are fatty foods, citrus fruits, milk and milk products, tomatoes, onions, pineapples, pork, and avocado. Whether these foods actually trigger migraine and the mechanism by which they do so remain to be scientifically documented.

Medications

Certain medications are capable of producing headaches, particularly in those people predisposed to migraine. Among these agents are reserpine, oral contraceptives, blood-vessel dilating drugs such as nitroglycerine, hydralazine, some diuretics (''water pills''), and anti-asthma medications such as aminophyllin.

In addition to these agents, prolonged use and subsequent and sudden withdrawal from ergotamine, amphetamines, propranolol, and phenothiazine drugs may provoke a vascular headache. Ergotamine withdrawal headache (rebound) is discussed in Chapters 7 and 18.

Atmospheric Weather Changes

Many individuals identify changes in weather as having a provoking influence on their migraine attacks. During the past several years, attention has been focused upon the relationship between atmospheric weather changes, air ions, and biological disturbances. Air ions are electrically charged air particles, the ratio of which varies with changes in weather and air pollution among other factors. They are thought to exert an influence over body physiology. The ill winds throughout the world, which include such entities as the Argentina *Zonda*, Mediterranean *Sirocco*, southern California's Santa Ana, Switzerland's *Foehn*, and Arizona's desert winds, are known for their ability to cause illness.

Researchers in Israel studied several hundred patients experiencing physical and mental discomfort with changes in weather brought about by the *Sharav* (dry heat) and *Bora* (cold rainy weather) in the Middle East. Among the many symptoms noted in this population were mental changes including malaise, irritability, and depression. Physiological discomfort such as generalized weakness was also seen. This study concluded that clinical symptoms correlated well with changes in body chemistry such as alterations in serotonin, thyroxin, steroid, and amine metabolism. Although many possible explanations exist, alterations in the ratio of positive to negative air ions which accompany these climatic changes are thought to be responsible for the physiological disturbances.

Understandably, this issue is unresolved. As with many issues related to migraine, there are differences of opinion. Work in the area of atmospheric events and body function is important, but no certain conclusions regarding a relationship between these changes and headache precipitation can be made at this time.

Other Provoking Factors

There are numerous other provoking influences for migraine. Sunlight and flickering or dazzling phenomena may trigger an attack in some individuals. It has been demonstrated that vascular headache provocation was brought about by sunlight in up to 30% of patients. The researchers who performed this study proposed that sunlight aggravated a preexisting brain excitability leading to excessive response of the blood vessels to stimulation.

Many patients report that their headaches occur during or soon after flying in airplanes. Pressurization changes, anxiety and "letdown," and the general turmoil of travel may account for some of these. In addition, those who travel long distances across various time zones may experience several days of headaches as a consequence of disturbed sleep/wakefulness cycles and the physiological consequences (jet lag). Some "holiday migraines" may be attributable to this phenomenon.

In later sections of this book, migraine-like headaches provoked by trauma, exertion, and disorders of the neck will be discussed. Likewise, several other medical disorders which may produce headaches similar to migraine will be detailed.

Summing Up

Many physiological and emotional events can serve to provoke a migraine attack, or at least a headache that is similar to migraine. Substantial disagreement exists among authorities regarding the reliability and validity of many of these influences. Generally, it is acknowledged that those predisposed to chronic headache, particularly the vascular headache disorders such as migraine, are more susceptible to these provoking influences. The exact relationship between them and headache, however, is poorly understood. Individual vulnerability varies greatly. Susceptibility appears to change periodically and during an individual's lifetime, and additive or cumulative influences may be necessary to provoke an attack. The inconsistent and variable effect of these factors and their inherent complexity makes migraine difficult to understand and explain and leaves ample room for legitimate differences of opinion.

6

Cause of Migraine

Though an old illness, migraine remains poorly understood. The actual cause of the disturbance cannot be described with certainty. This chapter will briefly review some of the important changes in our concept of migraine.

Since the 17th century, physicians have presumed that migraine is essentially caused by changes in the size of blood vessels. When the blood vessels narrowed (constricted), neurological symptoms would result. When the blood vessels expanded (dilated), throbbing and pounding headache occurred.

It is now clear that constriction and dilation alone cannot explain the pain or other symptoms of migraine. Medical research is now focusing on a variety of disturbances within the brain itself. These alterations in cerebral (brain) function are believed to underlie the blood vessel abnormalities and many of the other symptoms of migraine. Of primary importance in this changing attitude is the growing recognition of the role of that part of the brain called the hypothalamus. The hypothalamus is located behind the eyes and above the pituitary gland. It receives information from the parts of the brain that control emotions (the limbic centers) and communicates information to the pituitary gland, which is responsible for the control of many bodily processes, including hormonal changes. Among the many functions of the hypothalamus are control over body cycles, appetite, sleep, hormonal secretion, and the timing of many periodic body events such as menstrual periods, sleeping cycles, and hundreds of others.

The hypothalamus also communicates with the brain stem, the stalk of the brain which connects the two cerebral hemispheres to the spinal cord. This portion of the brain is now known to contain a very important "antipain" system that inhibits the body's ability to perceive incoming adverse stimulation as painful. Specialists in pain now believe that an interplay between pain perception and this antipain system in the brain stem is necessary for what is called normal pain modulation. Moreover, these systems must rely on certain neurotransmitters including endorphins, noradrenaline, and serotonin. Therefore inherited or acquired abnormalities in the production or function of these neurotransmitters may lead to disturbances that produce painful events such as migraine.

In this regard it is interesting to note that these same neurotransmitters are related to other disturbances frequently encountered in patients with headaches, including depression, family history of depression, sleep disturbances, and perhaps even tendencies toward alcoholism or medication overuse such as narcotic dependency.

Consider serotonin, for example. It is now known that the level of serotonin in the body falls dramatically prior to a migraine attack. Some researchers believe that this drop in serotonin levels results in the changing mood (often depression) that occurs just before or during a migraine attack. Serotonin has been pinpointed as being an important chemical factor in inherited depression.

Another line of thinking has to do with hypothalamic control over body cycles. Many researchers are coming to believe that intermittent rather than continuous disturbances of the hypothalamus are involved in the symptoms that are components of the migraine attack, including pain. Many now believe that these disturbances occur in cycles. This would explain why migraine may be present for a while, then absent for a while, with attacks returning unexpectedly for no apparent reason for them.

One of the recent discoveries is that for many patients, the "headache life cycle" begins with periodic occasional migraine. Over the course of the next 10 to 20 years, though (usually in their twenties or thirties), they begin to experience daily headaches with attendant overuse of painkillers, growing depression, and sleep disturbance. Many researchers now believe that this progression is more likely to occur in certain individuals with hereditary headaches.

In summary, the cause of migraine is not known, but researchers are no longer placing their primary focus on the blood vessels. Instead, they are paying more attention to the centers of the brain that control blood vessels and many other body functions. Growing understanding of the chemistry of the brain, how it works, and how it affects mood, pain, and organ function is leading us to exciting discoveries and bringing us closer to a more complete understanding of migraine and its cause.

7

How Migraine Headache Is Treated

The treatment of headache, migraine or otherwise, should begin the moment a patient enters the doctor's office. Many people claim that the medical profession reacts differently to the complaint of headache and chronic pain than it does to other illnesses, although the merits of this claim cannot be addressed here. Clearly, though, it is important for doctors consulted by people with chronic headache to take the patient's problem seriously, to convey a sincere interest in the patient's distress, and to understand the patient as an individual. Establishing a worthwhile communication between physician and patient is a vital part of diagnosis and treatment.

It is essential that the professional treating a patient in

chronic pain demonstrate concern for the patient and provide an open avenue for communication. Social and emotional disruptions that accompany or promote the pain should be explored, and the physician should allow ample time for questions about the patient's distress and the planned diagnostic and treatment program. The physician's ability to enlist trust, allay anxiety and fear, and encourage cooperation is critical to a successful treatment program. The person, even more than the symptom, requires treatment in chronic and complex cases. In the same sense, the patient needs to be open, honest, candid, and as helpful as possible.

Because current evidence suggests that migraine, and perhaps other chronic headache disorders as well, represent the physical expression of a genetically determined physiological predisposition, successful teatment should be directed at control rather than cure. In this regard, the treatment approach must draw attention to three therapeutic goals: 1) removing or modifying provoking influences, 2) controlling (to whatever extent possible) the exaggerated biological responsiveness, and 3) relieving the pain once manifest if it cannot be prevented successfully.

Despite claims to the contrary, there unfortunately exists no absolute cure for most recurring headaches. Most patients who have troublesome headache problems will not find simple solutions. Nonetheless, a variety of therapies, with and without medication, are available either to help avert the headache attack and prevent it from occurring or to reverse it, or at least lessen its intensity when it arrives. It is now estimated that up to 75 to 85% of patients with recurring headaches can receive substantial overall relief when properly treated.

Nonmedical Treatment

Whenever possible, physician and patient should try to relieve or prevent the headache attacks by nonmedical means—without drugs. I fully acknowledge the usefulness of many nondrug efforts and recommend them readily. Still, it seems clear that the most satisfactory outcome in many if not most headache patients still requires the use of medication, at least temporarily. This is particularly true to relieve the acute attack of migraine, in which medication above all other therapies is the most effective means of pain alleviation.

Controlling Provoking (Triggering) Factors In Chapter 5 the many influences that trigger migraine were discussed. The psychological and physiological events may act independently, together, or in concert with additional, yet unidentified, events to precipitate an attack. Isolation (and possible modification or even removal) of these factors represents a most important element in the treatment of a patient with migraine.

Emotional Factors Emotional factors are important in the precipitation of many migraine attacks. Prolonged stress, internalized anger and repressed hostilities, depression, and a wide variety of other emotional and personality issues influence headache and perhaps general health as well. Chapters 12 and 15 to 17 review various psychological aspects and several treatment approaches to these problems in headache patients. Although many patients with migraine demonstrate a variety of psychologically distressful features, these patients may be no more likely to carry these burdens than individuals not experiencing headaches. It is perhaps their biological predispositions, not their exact psychological nature, that render them vulnerable to a variety of headache-aggravating factors, not the least of which are psychological stresses. When stressful personality and psychological dynamics are present in someone predisposed to headache, persistent provocation may occur.

Dietary Control In Chapter 5 the possible relationship between dietary factors and eating patterns and the development of headache was discussed. The important question here is to what extent dietary manipulation should be employed. It is recommended that all patients with frequent headaches avoid long gaps between meals. Four to five well-spaced meals should be consumed daily. In addition, individuals with frequent headaches should avoid foods that contain tyramine, monosodium glutamate, milk products, and nitrite. This requires elimination of aged cheeses, chocolate, chicken livers, broad beans, and many processed foods. When feeling better, independent of what treatment program is employed (medical, nonmedical, or both), the patient can try gradually reinstituting one food group at a time.

An alternative approach is to place less emphasis on dietary manipulation until other treatments have been tried. For some patients, restricting diet or regulating eating habits is difficult and impractical. In others, it is preferable.

The role of diet in provoking migraine remains a matter of debate. It is likely that only a few patients will experience dramatic results from dietary manipulation alone. Nevertheless, the physician will occasionally encounter the patient in whom dietary factors play such a critical role in headache provocation that successful control of headache requires strict adherence to special diets.

Hormones and Other Drugs In Chapter 5, the aggravating role of homones in the development of headache was discussed. Oral contraceptives and supplemental or replacement estrogens should be avoided whenever possible. Occasionally, the administration of estrogens may prove beneficial in those with recurring headaches, but this is generally the exception rather than the rule.

When oral contraceptives or estrogen replacement is discontinued in an attempt to bring headache relief, beneficial results may not take place for several months. Headaches may seem to worsen during the first several weeks or months after discontinuance.

Hormones are not the only drugs that may trigger or aggravate migraine in general or in certain individuals. Among drugs that have been found to have such effects in some studies are various drugs used by people with arthritis or cardiac (heart) problems, drugs used to control appetite, some types of diuretics ("water pills"), medications used to control asthma, and even vitamins. This is why it is so important for the physician to take a careful history. It is equally important for the patient with migraine to inform the physician about *all* drugs he or she is taking, including so-called over-the-counter (OTC) preparations like aspirin, cold medications, and vitamin and mineral supplements. The physician may want to adjust the dosage, or it may be necessary to substitute a different medication or to discontinue the drug.

Maintaining Consistency in Daily Activities During the past several years, researchers have begun to investigate the importance of keeping to a consistent schedule for physiologically important events. Such regularity is being recognized as possibly helpful for patients with recurring headaches. For example, people with migraine are best advised to avoid disruptions in usual sleeping patterns. Sleeping extra hours on weekends and napping can provoke headache. Likewise, headache may occur if sleep time is shortened. Maintaining regular sleeping hours and avoiding extra sleep is useful. Suggestions for regulating your daily activities include:

- Try to get up and go to bed at approximately the same times each day, even on weekends or on vacations. Consistently awakening at the same time each day appears particularly important. ''Sleeping in'' and napping should be avoided.
- Try to eat at approximately the same time each day. Whenever you can, avoid delays between meals or periods of prolonged fasting.
- Try to pace your daily physical and emotional activities to a reasonable and consistent pattern. On weekends and holidays, begin the day approximately as though you were beginning the average day, pacing yourself as evenly as possible.

Correcting Existing Health Problems A variety of other steps may prove helpful. Your physician will be working with you to correct any physical abnormalities such as high blood pressure (hypertension), heart disease, or blood sugar (glucose) disorders, which might be contributing to your headaches. Consultation with a dentist may be helpful in ruling out tooth or serious jaw disorders.

Smoking Increasing evidence points to a link between headache provocation and cigarette smoking. Discontinuing or at least cutting down on smoking may significantly reduce the frequency of your headaches or may at least diminish their severity. I suggest that all patients with recurring headaches would be best served by discontinuing smoking as soon as possible. Some research suggests that the reason why smoking triggers or aggravates headaches is related to the harmful influence of both nicotine and carbon monoxide on the biological mechanisms of the brain.

Dependence on Painkilling Drugs It is now clear that the daily use of analgesics (pain killers) or certain other drugs for the treatment of headache can in many individuals aggravate and enhance the likelihood of recurring headache events. The overuse of such drugs as specific migraine agents (Cafergot, Wigraine, Ergostat), decongestants and nasal sprays, and simple over-the-counter analgesics may all cause a process referred to as *rebounding*. The rebound process reflects a subtle dependency on the drug, and discontinuance is essential if headache control is to be realized. Research is now pointing to the likelihood that increasing use of these medications stimulates a worsening of the headache process. Although these medicines do not initially "cause" the headache, over time they may become the fuel that ignites the next headache, resulting in an increasing cycle of pain and drug usage. Only by complete discontinuance of these agents, and the resulting "withdrawal period," can improvement occur.

Many patients have told me that it is only after they have stopped their excessive use of painkillers (Excedrin, Vanquish, Anacin, and others, including prescription drugs) that their headaches came under reasonable control either spontaneously or with the help of prescribed preventive medication that previously had failed to bring any relief.

Exercise and Relaxation Regular exercise, including jogging, swimming, bicycling, tennis, and racketball, and adequate relaxation are recommended. Exercise may have substantial value for some people.

Laughter is yet another self-help tool. A growing number of health professionals believe that laughter may have an important effect on the brain and thus on mental health. There is little doubt that laughter is a neurological event that integrates emotional and biological phenomena. Few of us would deny that there is something very special about laughter. After all, healthy laughter is contagious, it weakens the arms and legs by diminishing muscle tension, and it tends to produce a relaxing and almost soothing effect on emotions. Have you ever tried to be angry at someone who makes you laugh?

Some pain specialists, as well as the general public, believe that frequent laughter, high spirits, and joviality may actually bring about an improvement in pain and mental dynamics. I recommend to our patients that they learn to laugh each day, to let go of anger and memories of failures and losses, and to greet life with as much hope, lightheartedness, and optimism as possible. I fully recognize that this is not always easily achieved, but making a special effort at looking at the lighthearted side of life, and going about the process of finding something to laugh at heartily each day may be far more beneficial for headaches than would otherwise seem likely.

Biofeedback and Behavioral Therapy can be very helpful to many people with headache, including migraine. This subject is fully covered in Chapters 16 and 17. **Acupuncture** is reported to be temporarily effective, but it rarely works beyond the acute event, if it works then. Sustained benefit has not been scientifically demonstrated.

A word about **chiropractic** is necessary. Many patients with headaches have been told that their headaches are caused by abnormal conditions of their cervical spine (neck), including various types of dislocations. Most medical doctors, including myself, do not believe this to be true. Reviews of x-ray studies have failed to substantiate these claims. Although temporary relief of some types of headaches can occur with various types of massage and manipulation, longstanding relief is rarely forthcoming. Moreover, there are serious risks to aggressive manipulation. First, prolonged nonmedical therapy may delay proper diagnosis. In addition, manipulation itself has been documented to cause strokes in certain individuals. These comments should not be interpreted as suggesting that all chiropractic manipulation is imminently dangerous, but they should alert you to the fact that cervical manipulation has caused stroke and other serious neurological consequences in a small but important number of individuals who have been treated in this way. Do not assume that this or any therapy, medical or otherwise, is without potential risks.

Medical Management of Migraine

There are two basic approaches to medical treatment of any illness, including migraine: the *symptomatic approach* and the *preventive approach*. As the name implies, symptomatic therapies for migraine relieve pain that is evolving or already present. Some physicians refer to this approach as "rescue or reversal treatment." Preventive therapy attempts to forestall the migraine process. It is generally used for patients whose frequency of headaches has been increasing, for those who should not take symptomatic medications for some reason, or for patients whose headaches do not have a predictable pattern or do not respond to symptomatic measures.

The symptomatic and preventive approaches may also be

combined. Which approach your physician will use depends on a number of factors including the frequency, intensity, and duration of your headaches and your overall health profile. The doctor will also take your lifestyle into consideration and will evaluate your ability to follow a prescribed regimen. Factors involved in selecting a treatment regimen are listed in Table 3.

TABLE 3

Factors the Physician Considers in Choosing a Migraine Therapy

---

Symptomatic (rescue) therapy is used when:

- Headaches have a frequency of one or two per week

- Certain health problems that make certain medications inadvisable; for example:

  Patients with coronary artery disease, severe high blood pressure, and various blood-vessel disorders should avoid ergot derivatives, which tend to constrict the blood vessels

  Patients with peptic ulcer disease, using anticoagulant (blood-thinning) drugs, have aspirin-sensitive asthma, and some other conditions should avoid use of painkillers that contain aspirin

Preventive therapy is used when:

- Frequency of headache is greater than 1 or 2 headaches a week

- Medical conditions (see above) are present that make symptomatic therapies inadvisable

- Failure of symptomatic therapies is present

- A realiably predictable pattern of migraine attacks—for example, at or around the menstrual period—is present

- A known tendency toward substance abuse overuse exists

The Symptomatic Approach Symptomatic treatment of migraine is considered when headaches occur infrequently and medications used for this approach are acceptable in terms of the patient's health. The form in which a drug is given may be as critical as the choice of medication. Most medications for headache are administered in tablet form which makes the rate of gastrointestinal absorption a critical factor in the ultimate effectiveness of the drug.

In a study with important implications, a delay of stomach absorption was demonstrated in patients during both the acute phases of migraine and the preheadache aura. This delay was noted even in the absence of nausea and vomiting.

Even though delay may occur in many people during the acute attack of migraine, traditionally used medications given by mouth have proved valuable to a large number of migraine sufferers. These drugs should not be discarded simply on principle. If they fail to help, however, this may be related to a delay of absorption.

To stop a migraine once begun, the use of one or more medications is usually required. Although narcotic medications have a role in selected circumstances, the tendency for overuse and addiction to these medications by patients with recurring pain must be considered.

Ergotamine and Related Drugs For over 50 years, ergotamine tartrate has been the favored treatment for the acute attack. When given by injection, this drug is effective within an hour or two in 90% of patients. It takes effect within the same time span in 80% of patients when given in the form of rectal suppositories and in up to 50% of patients when given in pill form.

The exact mechanism by which ergotamine affects migraine is not known. It is believed to relate in part to the drug's constricting effect on blood vessels, but recent evidence suggests that it also might affect certain brain centers important in migraine. Ergotamine is available in a variety of forms that can be injected, inserted rectally, inhaled, swallowed, or dissolved under the tongue (sublingual administration). The oral and sublingual forms are not as effective as the injectable or rectally administered forms.

Ergotamine should not be taken by patients with high blood pressure, blood vessel disease, heart disease, certain medical illnesses such as lupus erythematosus, or patients over age 60. The drug must be used with great caution in the presence of significant peptic ulcer disease, slow heart rate, kidney or liver abnormalities, fever, or recent infection.

Like all medications, ergotamine tartrate may cause side effects. Among the minor reactions are nausea, vomiting, muscle aches, diarrhea, and a sense of difficulty swallowing. Though troublesome to many individuals, they are generally without serious consequence. The nausea probably occurs because ergotamine stimulates the brain's center for nausea, not because of any direct effect on the stomach. In addition, abdominal cramps, chest pain, a sensation of spinning, and tingling of the hands and feet are estimated to occur in 5 to 10% of individuals taking this drug. The most serious consequences of usage occur when excessive dosages are employed or when the drug is used in individuals who should not take the medication, although severe reactions have been reported at acceptable dosages and in otherwise healthy patients. Severe elevations of blood pressure, heart pain, and constriction of blood vessels to the arms and legs have been noted.

Ergotism is a serious consequence of prolonged overuse of this drug. It results in progressive nausea and vomiting; constriction of the blood vessels in the hands, arms, legs, and organs; mental changes; and other problems. This consequence of ergot usage is extremely rare and can be avoided by restricting usage to no more than twice a week.

Recently, an additional consequence of excessive usage of this drug has been noted. I and my colleagues have reported many patients in whom the recurring usage of ergotamine has led to an increasing headache pattern with resulting addiction to the drug and untreatable headaches. This process can be alleviated only by absolute elimination of all ergotamine usage, and frequently this requires hospitalization to achieve. It is my opinion that ergotamine should not be used more than twice a week, no matter how bad the headaches may be.

Though the comments on this drug might seem frightening, ergotamine represents one of the most effective and widely used drugs in the symptomatic treatment of migraine. It is still considered the "drug of choice," a phrase physicians use to describe their preferred drug for a given condition. When used carefully and in appropriate settings, this drug may bring dramatic relief to headaches that would otherwise seem untreatable.

Midrin Midrin contains no ergotamine. This preparation combines a mild vasoconstrictor drug that slightly narrows the blood vessels (isometheptane mucate), a painkilling drug (acetaminophen, the same drug as Tylenol), and a mild tranquilizer (trichlorphenazone). It exerts a beneficial effect on acute attacks of migraine and is used for mild to moderate attacks. It may produce less gastrointestinal distress than ergotamine preparations. Midrin is an excellent drug for moderately painful migraines. It may produce side effects such as mild sedation or light-headedness. Sometimes mild gastrointestinal distress is reported. All in all, however, Midrin is well tolerated by most patients with only a minimum number of side effects.

Analgesics (Pain Relievers) Although analgesics may benefit some people during an acute attack, the overuse of painkillers is a serious problem among headache sufferers. There are many medications on the market that can be used to relieve pain. Most of the over-the-counter medications contain aspirin, acetaminophen, and caffeine in various combinations. Some are just plain aspirin, and others, such as various forms of Tylenol, are primarily acetaminophen. Table 4 lists the various ingredients in popular over-the-counter as well as prescription preparations.

TABLE 4

Active Ingredients in Nonprescription Analgesics and Related Drugs

	Aspirin	Acetamino-phen	Caffeine	Other
Plain Aspirin	300–325mg	—	—	—
Tylenol	—	325mg	—	—
Extra Strength Tylenol	—	500mg	—	—

	Aspirin	Acetamino-phen	Caffeine	Other
Datril E.S.	——	500mg	——	——
Excedrin PM	——	500mg	——	mild sedative
Extra Strength Excedrin	——	500mg	65mg	——
Bufferin	325	——	——	——
Anacin	400	——	32	——
Anacin III	——	325	——	——
Percogesic	——	325mg	——	mild sedative
Cope	421	——	32	antacids
Vanquish	227	194	33	antacids
Midol	454	——	32.4	mild sedative
Panodol	——	500	——	——
Advil	——	——	——	200mg ibuprofen
Maximum Strength Anacin	500mg	——	32	——

	Aspirin	Acetamino-phen	Caffeine	Other
Maximum Strength Anacin III	——	500mg	——	——
Ecotrin	325	——	——	——
Maximum Strength Ecotrin	500	——	——	——
Nuprin	——	——	——	200 mg ibuprofen

Many headache centers will encourage patients not to use analgesics except for occasional headaches because of a process called ''rebounding.'' In this syndrome, the increasing use of painkillers actually fuels an increasing number of headaches until the headaches combine with overuse of painkillers to create a major problem. Discontinuing excessive or daily use of painkillers can relieve headaches, ironically, but many people with headache are afraid to give up their painkillers for fear they will experience increasingly painful attacks. The first several days after reducing painkiller overusage can be more painful than before, but over the period of days that follows, improvement is forthcoming. Sometimes a preventive (see later) program is used to help the patient during this withdrawal period.

Narcotics Injectable narcotics are of great value for some individuals, but the tendency for overuse must be emphasized. These medications should not be used as standard therapy during the acute attack since other less troublesome agents are available. Doctors have come to be concerned about patients who frequently seek narcotic analgesics for acute headache control. In time many of these patients become addicted to the treatment. Some of these patients may also be expressing through the vocabulary of pain deep-seated psychological neediness that must be met by other kinds of therapy.

Antinauseants and Other Medications Medications that counteract nausea can be very helpful in relieving the nausea that accompanies an acute migraine attack and sometimes in relieving the pain itself. They can also calm down the anxiety and jitteriness that accompany an acute migraine. A variety of medications are available for administration in tablet, suppository, or injection form. Suppositories are particularly useful because they need not be swallowed or digested by the stomach. The gastrointestinal distress that frequently accompanies a migraine attack causes problems with oral drugs. Other agents may also be effective in symptomatic treatment of headache. Hydroxazine (Vistaril, Atarax) given orally or by injection may also offer effective antinausea effects and may also relieve pain by itself or as an adjunct to other treatments.

Also effective are the nonsteroidal anti-inflammatory agents (the arthritis drugs), such as Motrin, Anaprox, Meclomen, and others. Sometimes these are used as preventives as well. Although propranolol (Inderal), nadolol (Corgard), and the tricyclic antidepressants (see below) are generally used to prevent headaches, some patients claim that taking them sometimes will help reverse a headache that has already begun.

A Warning About Symptomatic Methods As mentioned earlier, there are problems with symptomatic treatment of migraine. These rescue medications are generally safe and effective when used occasionally, but frequent use of certain of these can bring more problems than simply headache. Overuse of these symptomatic medications can intensify the frequency and the pain of migraine, causing a cycle to develop in which the medication itself becomes part of the problem (rebound effect). Discontinuance and withdrawal from these medications is often necessary in order to begin the process of relief. This problem is particularly likely with combination painkillers, particularly those that contain tranquilizers, as well as with ergotamine tartrate. Patients with frequent migraines (more than once or twice a week) should not rely on symptomatic therapies, because the likelihood of graduating to more frequent use during a difficult week or month is so great as to make the use of these agents undesirable.

Preventive Approach to Migraine

The preventive medical management of migraine employs the daily use of one or a combination of medications that are presumed to block the biological events leading up to a migraine attack. Your physician will consider such a program if your migraine attacks are so frequent that using symptomatic medications might be unsafe, if you have health problems that preclude using symptomatic drugs, or if your attacks follow a predictable pattern. Physicians usually begin a gradual reduction of preventive medication after three to six months of therapy. One reason for this is that natural remission of migraine does occur, and such a remission may not be recognized while the patient is taking preventive medications.

Many medications have been found useful in preventing migraine headaches. The most commonly used of these belong to three major classes of drugs: the beta blockers, the calcium channel blockers, and the tricyclic antidepressants.

A Word About Side Effects All drugs have potential side effects. In some ways, side effects indicate that the drug is working on various body functions. While uncomfortable or annoying side effects should be avoided when possible, they are not necessarily dangerous. Like all things in life, medical care requires some trade-offs. You and your physician must decide whether the benefit you may receive from any drug is worth enduring the side effects. The presence of side effect does not necessarily suggest that the drug should be reduced in dosage or stopped. Sometimes tolerance will occur over time. Bring all side effects to the attention of your physician and discuss with your doctor whether this indicates that discontinuance is appropriate or whether further use is acceptable.

The Beta Blockers The beta blocking drugs were first developed in the early 1960s. Inderal (propranolol), the first of these agents widely used for headaches, was initially discovered to be of benefit in controlling angina pectoris ("heart pain"). Over time, research demonstrated that beta blockers were also very useful in preventing migraines. The exact mechanism by which the beta blockers control headaches is not known, but effects on blood vessels or on brain centers is considered likely. In addition to Inderal, several other agents have been recently recognized as useful. These include nadolol (Corgard), Tenormin (timolol), and Lopressor (metoprolol).

Treatment with the beta blockers requires individual dosage determinations since people vary in their sensitivity in response to these agents. Short-acting and long-acting forms exist, so some are taken several times a day while others can be taken only once or twice a day. Therapy generally begins at the lower dosages with increasing dosage schedules over time. Reduction of blood pressure and pulse are common, so the physician must carefully monitor the patient while the correct dosage is being determined.

Most individuals taking the beta blockers will experience mild reduction in exercise tolerance, a sense of fatigue, and sometimes mild weight gain. Stomach or intestinal distress, reduction in sexual function, and sometimes even loss of hair are occasionally seen. These symptoms are reversible when the drugs are withdrawn or the dosages lowered. The beta blockers should not be given to patients with certain conditions including severe heart failure, severe low pressure, asthma, severe diabetes or severe hypoglycemia, or severe allergic conditions involving breathing problems. Some patients with depression may experience greater depression while on certain of these medicines, and other patients have reported mild reduction in memory.

Combining the beta blockers with certain diet-controlling medicines may be potentially harmful and should be done only with careful monitoring and under the guidance of a physician. Sudden discontinuance of these agents may bring about symptoms including rapid heartbeat (tachycardia) and changes in blood pressure. If the drug must be discontinued for any reason, it should be tapered off rather than being stopped abruptly.

The Calcium Channel Blockers During the past several years, a new group of medicines has made its way into the regimens prescribed for headache. These drugs, referred to as the calcium channel blockers or calcium antagonists, have a different effect from the beta blockers. Beta blockers tend to prevent blood vessels from dilating. Conversely, the calcium channel blockers open up certain blood vessel channels. They are called "blockers" because, ironically, they *open* blood vessels by *blocking* the flow of cellular calcium, which works to constrict blood vessels. The calcium channel blockers affect many other body systems, and some of them may affect certain brain functions as well. Research with calcium channel blockers suggests that they might be of benefit in chest pain (angina pectoris), certain circulatory problems, headache, certain digestive and gastrointestinal disturbances, and others.

Three major calcium channel blockers are available, each with a somewhat different mode of action. Your physician may prescribe one or another over a period of several months. These agents have relatively few side effects, but those that are common include increasing headache, dizziness, gastrointestinal distress, swelling of the ankles, and sometimes depression. These medicines can sometimes lower blood pressure and pulse rate as well.

The usefulness of calcium channel blockers in headache and specifically migraine has only recently been recognized. A full appreciation of their potential value awaits further experience. Like all medications, these drugs will not benefit all patients. The physician will generally start with low dosages and will then increase them over several weeks' time.

Because of the current interest in the relationship between body levels of calcium and maintaining bone strength, the name "calcium channel blocker" may promote worries about osteoporosis (bone deterioration) in patients who take them. It is important to emphasize that the calcium channel blockers do not affect blood calcium. They will not interefere with calcium metabolism of the kind important for bone strength.

Antidepressants The third major class of drugs useful in the prevention of migraine are the antidepressants. Currently, two major classes of drugs are available: the tricyclic antidepressants (TCA) and the monoamine oxidase (MAO) inhibitors. The tricyclic antidepressants have been known to be helpful in pain for the past ten years. Elavil or Endep (amitriptyline) is among the most important of these agents. The mechanism by which they help migraine is not known but is thought to involve their effect on raising certain levels of brain chemicals. Scores of tricyclic antidepressants are currently on the market, with many variations in side effects, speed of action, and other individual characteristics. For headache, many authorities have found amitriptyline (Endep, Elavil), nortriptyline (Aventyl, Pamelor), and doxepin (Sinequan, Adapin) most useful.

In addition to their value for headache, tricyclic antidepressants are frequently very helpful in sleep disturbances, which commonly accompany recurring headaches.

Common side effects of the tricyclic antidepressants include dry mouth, sedation, retention of urine, constipation, blurred visions, intense dreaming, weight gain, and lowering of blood pressure. They can worsen glaucoma and prostate disease. Many of these symptoms are dose related, and when the dosage is reduced the symptoms abate. These agents should not be used with severe heart rhythm disturbances, certain types of glaucoma, recent heart attack, epilepsy, or in conjunction with certain other medicines.

Tricyclic antidepressant therepy is sometimes combined with other preventive agents such as the beta blockers or calcium antagonists.

The monoamine oxidase inhibitors (MAOIs) represent the oldest class of antidepressants. More recently, they have come into popularity in the treatment of the more difficult headache conditions. Their use over the past 20 or 30 years has been minimized because of certain potentially serious side effects that can occur when these drugs are combined with certain dietary elements. It has also been considered dangerous to combine certain of these agents with the tricyclic antidepressants. During the past several years, however, first research centers and then practitioners have begun to combine these drugs carefully with good success. The MAO antidepressants should be used only under certain conditions, and only with specific guidance from physicians. When used carefully, however, they can provide a major control over certain types of migraine.

MAO inhibitors can cause lowering of blood pressure, dizziness, insomnia, reduction of sexual interest, and sometimes weight gain. These drugs, however, are particularly useful when severe depression and migraine coexist.

Sansert (Methysergide) Historically, the drug Sansert (methysergide) represented the primary agent for prevention of headaches. Sansert can be beneficial in up to 50 to 60% of migraine victims. The use of this drug, however, greatly diminished when beta blockers came onto the market. The exact mechanism by which this drug works is unknown, but an effect on blood vessels or certain brain cells is considered likely.

Adverse side effects of Sansert limit its usefulness. The most common of these include temporary muscle aching, abdominal, leg, or chest pain; hallucinations; and a sense of swelling of face or throat. With prolonged use (longer than six months without interruption), the drug has been known to promote the development of scar-like tissue in certain parts of the abdomen and chest. Many of these symptoms can be relieved by discontinuing the drug, but concern about these and other side effects including constriction of blood vessels, has limited the popularity of this very effective drug.

Physicians now use Sansert only under special circumstances and only in patients who are under 50. It should be given for only short periods (4–6 months) alternating with a period of at least one month when the drug is stopped completely. During this "rest" period the patient should have a chest x-ray and an x-ray study of the kidneys (intravenous pyelogram). When administration of Sansert is discontinued, it should be done by slowly reducing the dosage over several days to a week.

Tranquilizers Routine use of tranquilizers in treating migraine is not advisable, but some patients definitely benefit from occasional short-term use during periods of intense anxiety. The **benzodiazepine group** of medications (Valium, Xanax, Tranxene, Librium, Ativan, and others) are relatively safe, but can produce dependency with prolonged use. These agents may also increase depression, a common problem in certain anxious people. These drugs may have benefits in treating migraine beyond simple control of anxiety. They act on certain centers in the brain, which may explain why they sometimes help patients who are neither anxious nor tense. They also relax the muscles.

The stronger tranquilizers, those belonging to the group of medications known as the **phenothiazines,** have been traditionally used for serious mental illness such as schizophrenia. Their use in headache is limited, but some patients with complicated biological and emotional backgrounds have found that taking these drugs has some value, particularly for short-term use. Side effects are many, and prolonged use may bring about an uncontrollable movement of muscles in the face and elsewhere called *tardive dyskinesia*. Acute and sudden reactions involving tongue and throat are occasionally seen. This group of medications is particularly helpful in controlling nausea during acute migraine. They are usually quite safe when used in this way.

Cyprohepatadine (Periactin) has an antihistamine effect in addition to its tranquilizing properties, but its value in migraine is probably not related to its antihistamine features. This drug is not highly regarded for effectiveness in adults but is considered one of the best agents for preventing headaches in children. Periactin produces sleepiness, appetite increase, and dry mouth. It may aggravate epilepsy, certain types of glaucoma, certain gastrointestinal disturbances, and prostate disease.

Other Drugs Used in Preventive Therapy The **nonsteroidal anti-inflammatory** agents (the arthritis drugs) have already been discussed in terms of symptomatic use. They can also be used preventatively. These drugs are marketed under various trade names such as Anaprox, Meclomen, Motrin and Indocin. Each has different properties, and the physician must find the right drug for each patient. It may be necessary to try various drug groups to find the most effective preparation.

Major side effects include stomach distress (ulcer-type symptoms), swelling (edema), and sometimes lip sores. Most patients have no problems even with prolonged use, but careful monitoring for side effects is needed. Prolonged uninterrupted usage may damage the kidneys.

There are many other drugs that are useful in certain circumstances. These include Bellergal, certain anticonvulsant medicines (anti-epilepsy drugs) and others. **Bellergal** is a combination of ergotamine tartrate, a mild antinauseant, and a sedative (barbiturate). This drug's long-term use is discouraged because it can produce the "rebounding" problem previously described with ergotamine tartrate. Short-term use around the menstrual period can be of benefit.

A few patients who do not respond to traditional medicines will respond to the anticonvulsant medications, such as Dilantin (phenytoin) and Tegretol (carbamazepine). How these medicines work on migraine is not well understood.

Special Circumstances

Certain special circumstances require additional approaches. **Menstrual migraine,** which occurs just before, during, or after the onset of the period, is a difficult problem for some women. Most authorities believe that menstrual migraine results from a reduction in estrogen levels, which fall over the course of days preceding the period.

The headache associated with menstruation can be severe. Symptomatic as well as preventive medications are sometimes necessary. Occasionally, injections are required. Most patients with menstrual migraine can find relief with a combination of a preventive agent and a symptomatic agent given simultaneously. The nonsteroidal anti-inflammatory drugs, Bellergal, or others can sometimes be used preventively. Symptomatic treatments, including use of ergotamine tartrate, can help reverse the headache once it begins.

Some patients will have **prolonged intense headache** lasting not just a few days but sometimes weeks. A special form of ergotamine known as DHE (dihydroergotamine) has been given intravenously to reverse this type of attack. The intravenous administration of this medication, together with plenty of fluids, can terminate a prolonged period of headache that would not respond to conventional therapy. The use of cortisone-like drugs can also be of value for patients with this kind of headache.

Some patients simply cannot be helped by outpatient care, and **hospitalization** is sometimes required to provide control of headache, replenish fluids, and treat accompanying symptoms. In 1979, our center developed what was at that time the first hospital headache treatment unit in the world. This unit is now used for patients with especially severe problems, some of whom have been referred from around the world. Our program employs a special team of health professionals who aggressively and innovatively address the problem of headache control. The benefit from this and similar programs has been experienced by thousands of patients who have otherwise not found relief from their headaches.

8

Cluster Headaches

Following a period of perhaps several hours, during which I feel quite elated and energetic, I experience a fullness in my ears, somewhat more on the right side than on the left, having a character not unlike that which occurs during rapid descent in an airplane or elevator. I next become aware of a dull discomfort and extension of ear fullness in the base of my skull—further extending over the entire head, on both sides, although somewhat more on the right. At this point two or three minutes have elapsed, seemingly short but long enough for me to know that indeed a "cluster" has begun and will ultimately get worse. Such anticipation causes me considerable consternation regarding my decision to continue my activities or cancel plans and find a place to be alone; this gives way to a slowly increasing anxiety, fear, panic, and withdrawal. I become aware of myself "listening" to changes in my head. Is the cluster prematurely aborting itself, progressing further, or unchanging? A sudden stab, only fleeting, strikes my temple, then again— somewhere near the apex of my skull and upper molars in my face—always on the right side. It strikes me again, deep into the skull base and has quickly changed location to a small area above my eyebrow. My nose is stuffed yet runs simultaneously. If I could sneeze I feel the attack would end but in spite of all tricks I find myself unable to induce sneezing.

While the sharp stabs continue in this fashion, a slow crescendo of dull pain presents itself in an area of a hand's length and breadth over the eye and temporal region. The area of pain narrows into a smaller area but as if magnified enlarges in intensity. I find myself bending my neck downward, though slightly, as if my head were being gently pushed from behind. My neck, up in the base of my skull, is tight. It feels as if I were wearing a neck collar. I am compelled to remove my tie and loosen my shirt collar even though I know that it will not offer me even a modicum of relief.

In an attempt to alter this persistent discomfort, I drop my head between my legs while seated. My face and eyes seem to fill with fluid but the pain remains unchanged. In spite of my suntan, as I look into the mirror, a gaunt, sickly pale face peers back. My right eyelid is only slightly drooping and the white of my eye is charted with many red vessels, giving it an overall color of pink.

Having difficulty standing in one place too long, I leave the mirror to continue my alternating pacing and sitting.

As usual, I am struck with the additional fear that the pain will never end, but I dismiss it as impossible, since even if it were the case, I would surely kill myself.

The pain, now located somewhere behind my eye and slightly above, worsens. The pain is best described as a "force" pushing with such incredible power through my eye that my head appears to be moving backward, yielding its resistance. The "force" waxes and wanes, but the duration of successive exacerbation seems to increase. The cluster is at its peak, which is celebrated by an outpouring of tears from my right eye only. I have now been in cluster for 35 minutes—10 minutes at its peak.

My wife peeks into the room in which I hold the fort. I look up and see her expression of pity, frustration, and helplessness. She sees my tortured face as I have seen it in the mirror at this stage before; a drooling mouth, agape, gray face wet on one side, an almost closed eyelid, and swelling of pain and anguish. She closes the door and leaves, feeling hurt for me, anger for the stupidity of medical science, and guilt—since deep within her mind is the suspicion that she is the cause of my suffering.

I cry for her, but more for myself. The pain is so incredible. Suddenly I am overwhelmed by a fury. I lift a chair high above my head and crash it to the floor. With a doubled fist I strike the wall. The pain persists.

Waning periods soon become longer in duration and I allow myself to suspect that the peak is behind me—but cautiously, since I have been too often disappointed.

Indeed, the pain is ending. The descent from the mountain of pain is rapid. The "force" is gone. Only severe pain remains. My nose and eye continue to run. The road back, as with all travel, covers the same territory—but faster. Stabbing, easily tolerated pain is felt then gone. Dull, aching fullness, neck stiffness—all disappearing in turn, to be replaced by a welcome sensation of pins and needles over the right scalp area—not unlike after one's leg has been "asleep." Thus my head has awakened after a nightmare of torment.

Eye and nose dry, I let out a sigh. I collect my pile of wet tissues strewn all over the floor and deposit them in a waste paper basket. The innocent chair now uprighted, I rub my slightly bruised fist, having ended the battle and cleaned up its field, I open the door and enter my pain-free world—until tomorrow.

> Lee Kudrow, M.D.
> *Cluster Headache*
> Oxford University Press, 1980

The foregoing is a personal account of a cluster headache. The cluster headache is perhaps the most sinister of the well-recognized headache diseases. Few headaches surpass the ability of this disorder to cause panic, rage, and serious thoughts of self-destruction. And, few headaches more challenge a doctor's knowledge, compassion, and treatment skills than the cluster headache.

What is now called cluster headache has been known by many other names since the initial description by Dr. M. H. Romberg in 1840. Dr. A. P. Friedman and Dr. H. E. Mikropoulos helped firmly establish the term "cluster headache" after its clustering pattern had been described by Dr. E. C. Kunkle and others.

Types of Cluster Headaches

During the past several years numerous attempts have been made to reclassify cluster headaches in light of recently recognized variations from the classic patterns.

Episodic cluster headache is the most well known and most common pattern. It is characterized by recurring bouts or clusters of headaches, during which typical attacks (see below) occur regularly, usually daily. Each period or cluster lasts several weeks to several months, followed by a spontaneous remission lasting months to years. This remission is referred to as the *interim*.

Chronic cluster headache is subdivided into a *primary* chronic form and a *secondary* chronic form. The *primary chronic cluster* headache pattern is characterized by recurring headache events which, once they begin, undergo no periods of remission. The *secondary chronic cluster* headache is characterized by a pattern of typical, recurring headache attacks which have become chronic; they are unaccompanied by an interim, but have evolved from a previous episodic pattern. It is the absence of remission or interim for one year or more that justifies the term chronic in the primary chronic and secondary chronic forms.

Cluster migraine is a migraine-like headache syndrome with a periodicity similar to that of episodic cluster headaches, or in which cluster headache symptoms (see below) occur during otherwise typical migraine attacks.

Cluster vertigo is characterized by vertigo (severe spinning and loss of balance) during some or all otherwise typical cluster headache periods. The vertigo is not present during periods of remission.

Chronic paroxysmal hemicrania is a headache disorder with many similarities to cluster headache and considered by many to be a true variant. It is more fully described later in this chapter.

Signs and Symptoms

By contrast to migraine, a disorder that affects mostly women, cluster headache affects males primarily. The exact incidence of the disorder is not known, but it is estimated to afflict less than 1% of the population, from one-half million to two million people in the United States. The headache occurs in all major races and ethnic groups.

Cluster headache generally begins in the second or third decades of life, with a mean age of the late twenties. Onset after age 65 is not uncommon, nor is an onset earlier than 20 years of age. A 3-year-old child with symptoms similar to cluster headache from age 1 has been reported. The duration of the cluster period, that segment of time in the episodic syndrome during which attacks occur, ranges from 3 to 16 weeks. However, longer bouts may occur. The interim (period of remission) may last years but averages approximately 12 months.

During a cluster period, one or more attacks occur daily. Although the average frequency is one to three attacks per day, up to six attacks during a twenty-four hour period can occur. During the early or late phases in the cluster period, headaches may take place only a few days per week. Each attack lasts from 15 minutes to 2 hours, with residual discomfort for up to several hours after the termination of intense pain. A crescendo/descrescendo pattern is typical, evolving rather suddenly, reaching a peak, and terminating abruptly or more slowly. A headache may begin at any time of the day or night, and repetitive nocturnal awakening is very common. The adverse effect of sleep is shown by the likely provocation of daytime napping. Headaches occurring during sleeping hours are generally associated with rapid eye movement (REM) sleep.

The pain of cluster headache is extraordinarily distressing. Forceful, tortured, pressing, throbbing, burning, lancinating, seering, tearing, screwing, piercing, and stabbing are but a few of the descriptions used by patients. One patient described a red-hot iron being pressed into his forehead and eye until it had burned its way through his skull. Another characterized it as though the skin of his face and eyes were clawed away and acid poured into the open wound. One patient likened the attacks to a flame of a blow torch applied to his eye, while yet another described a burning metal spike being pounded through his eye and pushed into the skull.

Generally, the attacks are one-sided, usually around an eye, temple, or forehead. Those whose headaches focus on the eye socket or temple may report simultaneous pain in the neck or the base of the skull on the same side. A few people have experienced their primary pain location in the area where the head joins the neck, with only minor radiation to the temples or eye sockets. A substantial number of patients appear to experience pain in the lower half of the face. Radiation of pain into the jaw, nose, chin, and teeth is common. The headache typically strikes the same side of the head during each cluster period, but alteration of sides during different cluster periods is not uncommon.

Characteristically, the pain is accompanied by several additional symptoms and signs. Tearing of the eye on the same side as the head pain, in association with redness of the eyes and nasal stuffiness with drainage, is most common. Drooping of the eyelid on the affected side, pupil changes, unilateral or bilateral facial sweating, pulsating and tenderness of the blood vessels in the temple, and facial flushing are frequently seen. Enhanced sensory awareness and sensitivity to pain on the affected side are common. Preheadache symptoms and gastrointestinal distress as in migraine are relatively rare but have been reported. According to one researcher, another "associated finding" in cluster headache is the tendency of those experiencing an attack to pace, rock, or otherwise act out in anguish. In no other primary headache disorder is such behavior so typically exhibited.

A history of migraine is found in few male patients with cluster headache, but in many women. Occasionally, other family members will have cluster headaches. Those with cluster headache may say that cluster periods are reliably associated with certain seasons. Most studies, however, indicate that over time, attacks are equally distributed among all four seasons.

Like migraine, a cluster headache may be provoked by external stimuli—particularly alcohol. At least 50% and probably the majority of people with cluster headache are sensitive to alcohol during the cluster period. During the interim alcohol can be consumed without triggering headaches. Cluster headache patients, particularly men, possess a strong tendency to drink, even during a cluster period when headache provocation can be almost assured. Additional precipitating influences include cold wind or heat blown into the face, blood-vessel expanding substances in foods, especially nitrites, or in medication, letdown after work or excitement, and sleep.

Cluster headache may be associated with an increased likelihood of several illnesses, including peptic ulcer, coronary artery disease, and not unexpectedly, the consequences of alcohol abuse. An association with slow heart rate and low blood pressure has also been identified.

Other Diagnostic Clues

In the late 1960s, Dr. John Graham, a highly respected international authority on headache, first identified a particular facial appearance that occurred in many patients with cluster headache. He described this appearance as "lionized," which means lion-like. These men had very prominent skin lines, a thick-skinned appearance, and frequently a ruddy (reddened) facial skin.

Cluster headache patients tend to be taller than other men, are more likely to have hazel- or blue-colored eyes, and smoke heavily. They use alcohol to the point of abuse to a far greater extent than in the general population.

Biological Causes of Cluster Headaches

The cause of cluster headache is not known. Studies to determine the exact nature of this problem have not revealed definitive answers. What is proposed, however, is that the part of the brain called the hypothalamus is likely to be directly involved in cluster headache. The hypothalamus is the part of the brain that regulates body cycles, appetite, and hormone secretion; it links emotions with physiology. The idea of a hypothalamic origin for cluster headaches is supported by the cyclical pattern of the disorder. Why this area is abnormal is not known. The problem may be genetically determined or may result from trauma, internal body disturbances, or other factors.

Treatment of Cluster Headaches

Of all victims of chronic headache disorders, patients with cluster headache require diligence, innovation, and compassion—together with a firm knowledge of the relatively few tools available to curb the pain, desperation, and fear that afflict them. At our center at Ann Arbor, we make sure that patients requesting appointments are seen within a day or two, no matter how full the office schedule is. The choice is initial therapy must take into account the age and health of the patient, the frequency of the attacks, the expected duration of the cluster period, previous therapies, the patient's daily activities, and a variety of practical considerations.

Nondrug Aspects of Treatment Patients are strongly advised to discontinue all alcohol and to avoid daytime napping. If necessary, drug therapy is used to normalize sleep cycles. Patients are urged to stop or at least reduce cigarette smoking.

Inhalation of 100% oxygen is an effective means of symptomatically relieving the pain in many patients. Oxygen therapy must be begun early in the attack and a mask must be used to administer it.

Using Drugs to Treat Symptoms Aside from oxygen, effective symptomatic treatment of cluster headache generally requires the use of ergot drugs. If administered properly, ergotamine compounds are extraordinarily helpful in reversing most attacks within minutes. The limitation associated with the use of ergot preparations for cluster headache is that they will be required daily, thus exposing the person to the problems accompanying daily use of ergot alkaloids (see Chapters 7 and 18). Ergot preparations should be employed as a standby therapy for those attacks that could not be prevented (see below) or in circumstances in which no other effective means of control can be found.

Injectable narcotic painkillers are not advisable for the symptomatic treatment of cluster headache because of the tendency for overuse. Oral analgesics are usually without value, although over-the-counter sinus preparations have been preliminarily reported to help some patients. Daily, nonmonitored use of these agents poses considerable risk for abuse and adverse consequences.

Using Drugs in Preventive Treatment It is preferable to prevent cluster headaches instead of treating the symptoms alone, since the headaches occur daily during the cluster cycle. As in the preventive treatment of migraine, no medication can be consistently relied upon to provide effective pre-treatment.

During the past year or two, increasing attention has been paid to the usefulness of certain **calcium channel blockers** in the treatment of difficult-to-control cluster headaches. At our center we prefer the drug verapamil (Isoptin, Calan) although Procardia (nifedipine) and Cardizem (diltiazem) have helped some patients. The dosage of calcium channel blockers must be individually determined, using lower dosages initially and tapering upward to the point of effective control.

The use of **methysergide (Sansert)** was discussed in the chapter on migraine. It has a role in the treatment of cluster headache but should be used for only short periods and in only those patients in whom safety considerations have been taken into account.

Prednisone is a form of steroid (cortisone-like drug) and can be dramatically effective for short-term use. When given in sufficient dosage, it can effectively prevent up to 90% of cluster headaches. We provide a ten-day program of this medication and then follow through with another preventive medication. Prednisone dramatically reduces cluster headaches in most patients, making this a particularly useful drug for short-term use.

Because of its long-term side effects, which include reduction in immunity against infection, weight gain, ulcers, and aggravation of hypertension and diabetes, this agent is best used only for short periods.

Our center employs this drug for patients during "holidays" while they are off other medication, to obtain immediate relief for patients who are truly desperate, when patients are traveling, or when patients require an added "insurance" treatment for some reason.

This drug should not be used for prolonged periods, and should be generally tapered off rather than stopped suddenly.

Lithium carbonate (Eskalith, Lithobid, Lithane) was first reported effective in the treatment of cluster headache in 1974. Subsequently, it has been found to be very useful in up to 60% of cases. Lithium was first found useful in the treatment of manic depressive disease, a cyclical psychiatric disorder causing dramatic mood swings ranging from severe depression to hyperactivity and mania. The exact mechanism by which lithium helps cluster headache is not known but may in part be related to its effect on cycles controlled by the hypothalamus.

Lithium usage must be individualized, and lab tests should be done regularly to measure blood levels of the drug and various consequences of usage, including effects on the kidneys and thyroid. Side effects may include nausea, vomiting, diarrhea, tremor, blurred vision, unsteadiness, and aggravation of certain skin conditions, such as psoriasis. Patients using lithium must not avoid salt or take diuretics (water pills), because this can make lithium more toxic. Also, during hot summer months when salt depletion is common during periods of active perspiration, salt replacement or slight dosage reduction is sometimes necessary. Lithium can be combined with calcium channel blockers, and several other agents useful for cluster headache.

There are a large number of **other medications,** including the beta blockers, major tranquilizers, and nonsteroidal anti-inflammatory agents, which have been found useful in certain people with cluster headache. These can sometimes be combined with the major treatments listed above.

We have recently found that discontinuing smoking may also be useful for the treatment of cluster headache. Reducing smoking in some of our patients has been very difficult, but some who have done so have found their headache control to increase substantially. The patient must also avoid alcohol and other factors that aggravate headache.

Histamine desensitization is an old therapy, and certain authorities believe that it is still of value. This process requires hospitalization to desensitize the individual to histamine, and this requires intravenous injections. Most authorities do not believe that histamine desensitization is of value in most patients. Studies on allergy and headache have not established a close linkage to cluster headaches, and most authorities think there is no relationship between chronic recurring headaches and allergy.

Recently, certain surgical procedures have been found to help some patients with cluster headache. This treatment should be reserved for only the most difficult and hard to treat cases. It should not be used unless all other effective therapies have been tried and found ineffective.

Chronic Paroxysmal Hemicrania (CPH)

In 1974, Dr. O. Sjaastad and Dr. I. Dale described a new headache entity with a striking similarlity to cluster headaches. Although this disorder is quite similar to cluster headache, it possesses some distinctive differences. Chronic paroxysmal hemicrania primarily affects young women, though not exclusively. Although each attack bears a striking similarity to a typical cluster attack, headache events of chronic paroxysmal hemicrania may be shorter than those of a typical cluster headache. They generally occur with greater frequency, usually during the day, rarely awakening patients from sleep. Chronic paroxysmal hemicrania is almost invariably controlled by indomethacin (Indocin), a nonsteroidal anti-inflammatory drug.

9

Headaches Related to Muscle Contraction

William G. Speed III, M.D., F.A.C.P.

Currently, a major change in our understanding of headaches as they relate to muscle contraction is underway. Many specialists in headache disorders are coming to believe that the muscles are simply the victims of changes that are occurring in the brain. Some of the pain may come from muscles or may simply *appear* to be coming from muscles. While it is clear that some head and neck pain, particularly that involving the neck and shoulders, is of muscular origin, it is unclear why or how the process begins. Growing recognition of how the brain works and how headaches may be the consequences of the changes in the brain, is beginning to challenge the traditional viewpoint with respect to muscular relationship to headache. This chapter reflects our traditional theory on headaches as they relate and are caused by muscle contraction phenomena. This information will give you the proper perspective from which to judge the changing concepts as they become more apparent over the next several years.

How Muscular Contraction Is Related to Headache

About 90% of all headaches are related in some way to expansion of blood vessels (vascular dilatation) in the head, to contraction of certain muscle groups in the head and neck, or to a combination of these factors. Physicians have observed that excessive contraction, or tensing, of the muscles may be associated with pain. Testing of patients with a technique called electromyography (EMG) has confirmed this observation. An EMG utilizes electrical current to evaluate the contractile response of the muscles. Sometimes, though, pain is present at times when EMG studies do not show that excessive muscle contraction is present.

Possibly there are variations of contraction-related pain disorders in which excessive muscle contraction initiates pain that persists after the muscles have relaxed. We do know that voluntarily keeping muscles contracted for periods of longer than two minutes causes pain that may outlast the contraction itself. Therefore it is possible that patients who suffer chronic muscle-contraction headaches have periods of excessive muscle tensing alternating with periods when muscle tone, or state of contraction, is normal. If an EMG is done during this interval phase, it will not show any increase in muscle activity. Even so, muscle contraction may be the underlying cause of the patient's pain.

The Physical Mechanism of Contraction Headache

To understand how muscle contraction can cause headaches, one must have some understanding of how the nervous system regulates the contraction and relaxation of muscle tissue to keep the body upright and to initiate and control body motion. Special cells in the brain interact with motor neurons in the muscles and with nerve cells elsewhere in the body to regulate muscle tone. Any factor that has an adverse influence on any part of this maintenance system may cause it to exceed its limits; for example, it may result in excessive or overly sustained contraction of a muscle or system of muscles. This mechanism leads to pain, and the anxiety related to pain stimulates body mechanisms that create even greater tension in the muscles (the fight/flight reaction). Here you can see the self-sustaining cycle of events that we call chronic muscle contraction headache. Exactly how sustained muscle contraction causes pain is not known with certainty.

Types of Muscle Contraction Headaches

Like other illnesses, muscle contraction headaches may be classified as either acute or chronic. The acute type is quite common. The headaches are usually mild to moderate in intensity. They involve the sides and front of the head, the back of the head and neck, and the crown or top of the head, separately or in any combination. They are described as tight, pressing, squeezing, aching sensations and may be triggered by such things as fatigue, an acute family crisis, peaking of stressful work loads, or any other temporary stressful situation. They usually subside once the offending stimulus ceases, or they may be relieved by various over-the-counter analgesic pain remedies. Most people with the acute form tension headache do not seek the services of a physician.

Chronic muscle contraction headache, on the other hand, is constant and unremitting over weeks, months, years, or decades. The same areas of the head are involved as in the acute type. The characteristics of the pain are similar, but in addition patients with the chronic form of contraction headache describe soreness, weight-like sensations, tight bands, a feeling like that of a tight skullcap, and crawling sensations. Sometimes there may be intermittent jabbing, stabbing, or piercing components.

Some people with muscle contraction headache may also have associated vascular headaches which are described as throbbing and pounding. The intensity of the blood vessel–related headache component is aggravated by jarring the head, bending over, coughing, sneezing, and straining and by exposure to bright lights, loud noises, and physical exertion. The intensity of the muscle contraction component is not aggravated by these factors. In these patients it is possible that expansion of the blood vessels is a kind of rebound following the vasoconstriction that may be associated with muscle contraction. These headaches may also reflect concurrent attacks of migraine. The term "mixed type headache" is sometimes used to describe those headaches produced by a combination of muscle contraction and blood-vessel expansion (see Chapter 10).

Also like other kinds of illnesses, muscle contraction headaches may be primary or secondary. Among the underlying health problems that may lead to these headaches are eye problems including inflammation, muscle imbalance, or abnormalities of the visual process; inflammation of the nose or sinuses; disorders of the temporomandibular joint, or hinge of the jaw (TMJ pain); bone or muscle disorders of the neck; inflammation associated with a systemic infection such as a cold or flu; trauma (injury); tumors; or blood vessel dilatation. For the most part, however, muscle contraction headaches are not related to such physical abnormalities but rather to internal biological or emotional traits that produce tension, anxiety, or depression.

Some people with chronic muscle contraction headache may also have this problem because of injury to the greater occipital nerve, a nerve that runs up on either side behind the ear in the junction where the neck and head join. Injury to this nerve can occur from whiplash, falling to the ground and striking the back of the head, and similar accidents. Pain and tenderness frequently are felt at the base of the skull and can radiate forward to the top of the head or to an eye. The muscles around the area are frequently tight and restrict movement.

This condition is sometimes treated by injecting a local anesthetic to freeze the area, but pain relief may be short-lived. More permanent relief may result from surgically reducing the pressure on this nerve or even cutting parts of it. If the nerve itself is cut, permanent numbness of that area may result.

Often, the cause of chronic unremitting muscle contraction headaches is readily identified as being one of the conditions described above. Other cases are not so easily categorized. For example, some people with minimal anxiety or depression and no organic abnormality may have chronic muscle contraction headache. This suggests that in some individuals there is an intrinsic difference in biological responses which may cause muscular or neurologic mechanisms to be more sensitive to the usual stresses of life, perhaps inducing headaches, even though the stresses and ability to cope do not fall outside what would usually be considered normal. This difference may result from inborn variations in the sensitivity of the control mechanisms for muscle tone.

How Muscle Contraction Headaches Are Treated

Acute muscle contraction headaches subside when the offending stimulus ceases or is relieved by simple pain-relief medication. The person with chronic muscle contraction headache is not so easily treated.

How the physician approaches the chronic type of headache depends on the source of the muscle contraction. If it is secondary to problems of the eyes, nasal area, or jaw, or to brain disease, then specific treatment must be directed to these underlying problems. If there are underlying disorders of the neck (cervical spine), a nonsteroidal anti-inflammatory medication such as aspirin, indomethacin (Indocin), naproxen (Anaprox, Naprosyn), or ibuprofen (Motrin) might be tried.

Physical therapy may be helpful, including massage and even occasionally traction. Some individuals can use these therapies at home. Therapies such as standing in a warm or hot shower, massaging the scalp muscles, and the use of electrical stimulation with transneural stimulation units (TENS units) can be helpful at times.

Muscle contraction headaches that are secondary to inflammation resulting from medical disorders such as viral infections will subside with the termination of the viral illness. During the active phase, the muscle pains are usually eased by the use of aspirin, acetaminophen (Tylenol), or other mild analgesics.

When trauma is involved and the pain results from muscle contraction, the treatment is the same as that described for chronic muscle contraction headache unrelated to trauma. If there are associated areas of local tenderness, these are best treated with local anesthetics injected directly into the tender area.

When expansion of the blood vessel, such as occurs in migraine, is the primary cause of the headaches, there may be an associated contraction headache. In these circumstances, muscle contraction headache will usually subside once the blood-vessel problem is corrected.

What is left represents the vast majority of muscle contraction headache. When you first consult a physician about long-standing chronic muscle contraction headaches, it is important to tell him or her what medications you are taking, including over-the-counter drugs. Many patients who suffer continual headaches take large amounts of pain-relieving drugs and tend to become habituated to them even though they are producing little or no benefit. A growing number of researchers are suggesting that long-term use of analgesics may perpetuate chronic pain. For this reason, your physician may urge you to discontinue their use.

Tricyclic antidepressant compounds are the most useful drugs for treating chronic tension headaches. These compounds appear effective even if concurrent depressive symptoms are present, but we do not yet know exactly how they work.

Amitriptyline (Endep, Elavil) is the most effective of these compounds and can be given as a single dose at bedtime. A low dosage may be prescribed at first and may then be gradually raised as necessary. The maximum benefit may not be seen for two or three weeks.

Other drugs that your physician might consider include nortriptyline (Pamelor, Aventyl), desipramine (Norpramin, Pertofrane), or doxepin (Sinequan, Adapin). These drugs and their side effects were discussed in the chapter on migraine.

Sometimes beta blocking drugs or even the calcium

channel blockers are helpful, particularly when combined with the tricyclic antidepressants. Why this is so is not entirely clear, but mixtures of headaches may be present in a variety of different individuals and a primary influence on muscle contraction centers in the brain may result from the use of these other medical agents.

Muscle relaxants are usually not as effective as their name might suggest. Among the agents that can be useful in selected individuals are carisoprodol (Soma), cyclobenzaprine (Flexeril), orphenadrine (Norflex), and Skelaxin. Tranquilizers may be of limited value, although long-term usage must be discouraged.

Biofeedback can be of significant value in the management of muscle contraction headache, specifically if combined with EMG monitoring, feedback, and relaxation instructions (see Chapters 15 and 16). If this technique is to help you, you must be motivated ''to make it work'' and must be able to concentrate. The purpose of biofeedback is to train people to use their thought processes, consciously relaxing to override the physiological disturbance that produces muscle contraction headache. EMG monitoring helps them see when their muscles are contracting or relaxing. With good instruction and adequate practice, the biofeedback process itself may become more or less automatic. This is the ultimate goal for this therapeutic technique.

It is of utmost importance that you understand your headaches and recognize that you and your physician must work together to resolve your problem. Counseling may supplement biofeedback and medication. There is a generally accepted psychological mechanism by which emotional factors may precipitate muscle contraction headaches by translating anxiety into a physical symptom or a symbolic representation of psychiatric distress. The genesis of such anxiety may be deep-seated in earlier interpersonal conflicts, and therefore some patients with chronic muscle contraction headaches may need to consult a mental health professional. There are no published studies of the effectiveness of psychiatric treatment in chronic muscular headache.

Summing Up the Data

Excessive muscle contraction is a common cause of headache, often called "tension headaches." As the next chapter will suggest, though, our concepts of and attitudes toward the cause and treatment of these conditions are changing. The relationship between these headaches and tension, anxiety, and depression has been traditionally assumed, and it is no doubt relevant in many instances. Other factors, however, may be similarly or even more important, and these include various disturbances of brain centers that affect muscle contraction.

Because muscle contraction is often a response to underlying disorders, the physician will want to rule these out. Diseases that must be considered include disorders involving the eyes, nose, sinuses, temporomandibular joint (lower jaw), and various parts of the skull itself. Treatment generally requires individual considerations, and combinations of nonmedical therapies such as biofeedback and stress management, together with the use of certain medications (such as the tricyclic antidepressants) appear to help most patients.

10

Chronic Headache Complex: The Mixed Syndrome

Traditionally, migraine and muscle contraction headaches have been considered to be separate diseases. For this reason, and for convenience, they are discussed separately in this book. Actually, the situation is more complex than such classifications would suggest.

Traditional Assumptions About Headaches

To review what we have already discussed: Physicians do not yet understand exactly how migraine originates and progresses. Apparently, this kind of headache involves changes in the brain associated with changes in the blood vessels. Muscle contraction headaches ("tension head-aches") have traditionally been ascribed to painfully contracted muscles, although alternative theories have been advanced.

In terms of symptoms, headaches that are characterized by mild to moderate nonthrobbing pain or tightness in the region of the head and neck have been diagnosed as tension headaches. The assumption is that the brain, nervous system, and circulatory mechanisms are not primarily involved. The criteria for a diagnosis of tension headache have been so imprecise that this category has become a kind of diagnostic wastebasket to which physicians may tend to relegate any disorder that is clearly not vascular, is not identified with any underlying physical disorder, and includes elements of stress, anxiety, or depression.

Migraine as a separate entity has been discussed in earlier chapters. In Chapter 9, Dr. Speed explained the signs, symptoms, and bodily mechanisms associated with muscle contraction headaches. In this chapter we discuss a kind of mixed phenomenon in which migraine-type symptoms and those usually ascribed to muscle-related headaches coexist. They may occur together or at separate times.

Recent observations, however, provide additional considerations and new perspectives in our understanding of headache disorders. Many features of muscle contraction headache can be found in patients with migraine between acute attacks. Also, various substances that are thought to aggravate headache in migraine patients can actually cause headache in patients diagnosed as having muscle contraction pain. Certain changes in the bloodstream found in patients with migraine have also been found in patients who have so-called tension or muscle contraction headache.

Dr. Alvin Lake, author of the biofeedback chapter in this

book, has demonstrated in his research that biofeedback directed at muscles can actually benefit patients with migraine. Moreover, medications that are primarily directed at muscles have been found useful in people with migraine. These findings suggest that migraine and muscle contraction headache may be linked together in ways not previously recognized.

Features of the Mixed Headache

In reviewing the case histories of patients with mixed headache, I have found at least three important patterns:

The first pattern is characterized by headache attacks in which distinctive features of migraine predominate. These headaches occur periodically over many years of life, until they ultimately subside. Although most attacks are clearly migrainous, muscular elements may accompany the migraine attack or occasionally precede it.

A second pattern consists of predominantly muscular or muscular-like headache events, occurring periodically for hours to days (acute muscle contraction headache) or chronically. Occasionally, or more often, features traditionally ascribed to vascular headaches such as sensitivity to light, digestive symptoms, and blood vessel changes occur.

A third pattern, and one that is both fascinating and puzzling, is characterized by an evolution from clearly separate, episodic migraine attacks in earlier life to a pattern of relatively constant headache distress in later years. During this late phase the patient has daily or almost daily muscular or muscular-like headaches and less frequent vascular or migraine-like attacks. Usually, the migraine is less intense but not necessarily less frequent than in earlier years.

A closer look demonstrates that most patients so afflicted

are women whose migraine headaches usually began in childhood or adolescence and were occasional—often occurring around the menstrual period. The headache events were separated by headache-free days. Over time, "muscular" pain develops. Eventually, often during their thirties and forties, a continual discomfort of nonspecific or muscular-like pain evolves which is periodically associated with vascular headache attacks. The frequency of the vascular episodes ranges from one to two per week to one or less per month.

In addition, several other important features appear to characterize many of the patients experiencing this form of headache. Excessive analgesic use is common, and depressive and anxiety elements along with sleep disturbances are often present. A family history of depression, alcoholism, and headaches is frequently reported. Table 5 summarizes the features of this syndrome.

TABLE 5

Possible Features of the Chronic Headache Complex

Daily or almost daily headaches
Intermittent migrainous events
History of occasional migraine
Daily or almost daily analgesic use, often excessive
Depression/anxiety elements
Sleep disturbances
Family history of:
   headaches
   depression
   alcoholism

The mechanism of daily pain remains obscure. In some cases, muscular features such as band-like bilateral tightness or squeezing pressure are described. In others, however, the pain is characterized as a nonspecific Patients find it difficult to define. It is possible that, in some patients, this daily distress originates with a disturbance in the brain rather than in the muscles. It may also represent a natural transformation of migraine pain—or both mechanisms may be at work. I call this problem *chronic headache complex* (CHC) because it is chronic, headache is its most prominent feature, and it seems to originate from a combination of causative factors.

Treatment of Chronic Headache Complex

I have found that the simple mixed headache, in which both muscular as well as vascular features coexist during a well-circumscribed acute attack, is best treated with medications that relieve the kinds of symptoms that predominate. For acute migraine, ergotamine tartrate or Midrin, often in conjunction with drugs to counteract nausea, are appropriate. At times, medications useful for both elements are required.

The chronic headache complex is more difficult to treat. The patient must stop taking daily analgesics, preventive measures must be used, and appropriate social, family, and psychotherapeutic interventions are essential. Many patients must be hospitalized so that they can be weaned from analgesics and the biological and psychological factors of the disease can be dealt with. Medications most appropriate in preventing the headache include combinations of beta blockers and tricyclic antidepressants. Biofeedback is useful. Studies to further delineate this syndrome and its possible origins are under way.

11

Headaches in Children

Headaches do not spare children, and as in adults, the symptom of pain must be considered a possible indicator of serious disease. However, usually it is not. Beyond the medical issues, recurring and persistent pain in children has a heavy impact on family and social dynamics, threatening personality development and altering behavioral patterns. Ultimately, chronic pain in childhood can permanently affect the child's life and the way he or she relates to the world.

To complicate matters, some children with recurring head pain inevitably learn that painful suffering has a powerful influence over events. It may become a means of reducing their responsibilities, avoiding stressful confrontation, and enlisting more attention and love. Parental stress, often guilt and fear, in addition to school absences, altered family plans, and intensifying discord among family members are common.

Successful treatment of children with headache must encompass the entire family. It requires a broad understanding and sensitivity to family dynamics. Occasionally it also involves seeking the cooperation of school personnel. Repeated absences from school may prompt school authorities to take legal action against the parents, who may insist upon keeping the child home or retrieving the child from school during a headache.

The incidence of headache in children is not easily determined. Rates range from 2.5% of all children by age 7 to 18% of children between ages 10 and 12.

It is estimated that in 5% to 13% of all children experiencing chronic recurring headaches, serious illness or some medical or neurological problem is the cause. The majority appear to have migraine. Cluster headache is rare in children, but a variant, chronic paroxysmal hemicrania (see Chapter 8), is a childhood disorder.

This chapter explores chronic childhood headache syndromes. It is important to emphasize that children with headache, like adults, must be tested for minor as well as serious medical disease, which often mimic simpler and more benign headache conditions. Headaches may follow trauma in children just as they do in adults (see Chapter 13).

Childhood Migraine

Among adults, far more women than men suffer from migraine. In children the ratios are reversed; approximately 60% of children with migraine are male. In one study, children with headaches prior to 11 years of age were predominantly male, while those experiencing their first headache after age 11 were more likely female. Over 50% of children with migraine have a positive family history of headaches.

Symptoms of Childhood Migraine The onset of migraine in children has been reported as early as 12 to 18 months. Six years may be an average age of onset. Children with migraine may have symptoms similar to those of adults, but other symptomatic expressions, including migraine equivalents (see below), are also seen. In children experiencing adult-type migraine, both classic and common forms may be present. As in adults, common migraine occurs more frequently than classic. Although similarities exist between typical migraine of children and adulthood, there are differences, too. As already mentioned, boys are just slightly more likely to be affected than girls. Migraine attacks in children are apt to be shorter than those of adults, and gastrointestinal distress—especially vomiting—occurs more often. Throbbing pain, sensitivity to light (photosensitivity), and nausea and vomiting nearly always occur. Attacks may last from 30 minutes to several days. The triggering factors are generally similar to those in adults (see Chapter 5).

Vertebrobasilar migraine was described in Chapter 4. This type of migraine is common in children. The headaches are accompanied by signs of neurological involvement such as muscular incoordination (ataxia), partial paralysis on one side of the body (hemiparesis), vertigo, and alterations in consciousness. The child may become confused and may lose consciousness. These symptoms indicate neurological disturbances in the brain stem. Sometimes the neurological symptoms occur without accompanying headache. Children with vertebrobasilar migraine are likely to have a strong family history of migraine; that is, many other family members have been affected. Girls are affected more often than boys.

Childhood migraine may occur in the form of recurring paralysis, sensory abnormalities on one side of the body, and occasionally in speech difficulties (aphasia) together with the headache. These symptoms suggest that a disturbance in brain function and/or blood flow to the brain is involved. There may be a strong family history of similar attacks.

Migraine in children may also cause paralysis of the eye muscles, causing double vision. The pupils of the eyes may be enlarged.

Migraine Equivalents Migraine equivalents were described in Chapter 4. These symptom groups are sometimes called migraine variants. They often occur without an accompanying headache and are believed to reflect basic biological disturbances typical of individuals who are predisposed to migraine. Among the migraine equivalents are periodic irritability; recurrent attacks of vomiting, often with abdominal pain; episodes of dizziness and a spinning sensation (vertigo); periodic distortions of smell, vision, and body image; sleep disturbances; motion sickness; bedwetting; night terrors; and sleepwalking. *Episodic vertigo* takes the form of recurring episodes of spinning sensations. These are usually brief and are often accompanied by loss of balance and posture. Migraine equivalents occur most often between ages 2 and 4 but may also appear later. Children who eventually develop migraine have a higher rate of such disturbances than other children do.

Periodic vomiting, often accompanied by abdominal pain, fever, and headache, and usually lasting hours to days, is common in school-age children. Of children who have this problem, 75% later develop migraine. Excitement, stress, and anticipation are common provoking factors.

The relationship of migraine and epilepsy to periodic childhood syndromes is one of considerable controversy. The distinction between these disorders may not be obvious and is further confused by the occasional responsiveness of migraine, like epilepsy, to antiseizure medications.

Childhood migraine is triggered by the same precipitating events as adult migraine. Important factors include missing meals; sudden changes of lighting, such as when entering a bright area from a dark one; glare; and television and motion picture flickering. In addition, food sensitivity, physical exertion, automobile travel—particularly on bright sunny days, changes in weather, and head trauma are also common. Menarche (the beginning of the menstrual cycle at puberty) may bring with it the first migraine attack, as may a subsequent menstrual period (see Chapter 5).

Many attacks appear to occur independently of any apparent physical and psychological factor. They probably reflect internal changes in brain function.

Some authorities believe that children with migraine are more sensitive, neat, and tidy than others, and that they may be more easily frustrated. This theory has so far not been substantiated by research.

How Childhood Headaches Are Treated

Nonmedical (Nondrug) Treatment Although medications are useful and in fact essential to control some headache disorders of childhood, emphasis initially on nonmedicinal intervention is recommended. Stress issues are frequently present, often relating to family dynamics such as father/son and mother/daughter expectations, role playing, and school performance. Many youngsters with recurring headaches are timid, more sensitive than average, quiet and shy, creative, and apparently unable or unwilling to express their feelings openly. Childhood depression may take the form of headache.

Parents should be aware that behavioral therapy and biofeedback, together with family counseling and strategy development, have been used successfully to help children with headache disorders. It is important to consider these measures in conjunction with medical treatments. Intensive psychological counseling is occasionally necessary. (Biofeedback and behavioral therapies are discussed in Chapters 15 and 16.) Avoiding triggering factors, sleeping regular hours, getting up at the same time each day, avoiding junk food, and not missing meals must all be tried.

Medical Treatment A number of medications have proved useful in treating the symptoms of childhood headache disorders. Analgesics such as acetaminophen (Tylenol) may be given by mouth in tablet or liquid form or may be administered in the form of rectal suppositories. A word of caution about giving aspirin products to children: these drugs have been associated with a sometimes fatal disease known as Reye's syndrome in preteen children. The disease is characterized by damage to the liver and the brain, and it may be accompanied or heralded by a headache. More remains to be learned about the possible relationship of aspirin and Reye's syndrome, but meanwhile it might be best to avoid using aspirin products (see Table 4) for children with headaches.

Nausea can be relieved by medication, and barbiturates may also be used during acute attacks. Midrin or ergotamine tartrate may be employed when necessary.

Although symptomatic treatment is likely to be needed, preventive measures should also be tried, especially because recurring headaches are so detrimental to school attendance and may affect personality development. While these measures are being employed, an attempt should be made to reestablish normal living patterns.

Cyproheptadine (Periactin) is the drug most often used by physicians to prevent childhood migraine. Major side effects include mild sleepiness and increased appetite. This drug is discussed more completely in Chapter 7. Beta blockers may also be used. Antiseizure medications such as phenytoin (Dilantin) and phenobarbital are not generally beneficial to adults, but they may help children—especially those with vertebrobasilar migraine.

The antidepressant amitriptyline (Elavil, Endep) is also effective for some children, especially those who have mixed-headache syndrome or muscle contraction (tension) headaches. These drugs are best used in combination with other medications. Recently, the calcium channel blockers discussed in Chapter 7 have been found helpful for some cases of childhood migraine.

Summing Up

Watching one's child suffer is disturbing and anxiety provoking. The outlook for children with migraine is hopeful, however, especially for boys. Follow-up studies indicate that headaches cease totally in about one-third of affected children, and many others show marked improvement. The less favorable outlook for girls, reflected in the preponderance of women among adult migraine victims, suggests that the female hormone estrogen may be a triggering influence or a predisposing factor in migraine.

12

Headaches
Primarily Related to
Emotional Factors

Many chronic headache disorders are believed to reflect the body's biological overreaction to environmental stresses. However, emotions are a factor in many headaches. Stress, anger, rage, and "letdown" are a few well-known triggers of migraine and tension headaches. Even cluster headaches may be influenced by adverse or stressful emotional experiences, though less so than other forms of headache.

From this perspective, virtually all forms of chronic headaches could be called psychosomatic. That is, the biological mechanisms of the body (the *soma*) are influenced by the state of the *psyche*, or mind. Many health problems are known to be psychophysiological—that is, to have psychosomatic origins. Some of these diseases, which may be serious and even fatal, include colitis, peptic ulcer disease, asthma, and certain irregularities of heart rhythm. To this list we can add headaches. No matter what organ system is involved, brain and body are linked by a complex system of nerves and hormones, including the neurotransmitting chemicals that have been the subject of much recent research.

To convince yourself of the interrelationship of mind and body, think of the following circumstances in which thoughts lead to body change: tearing when thinking of a sad story, turning pale when frightened, turning red when blushing at an embarrassment, or feeling "goose bumps" when thinking about fingernails scratching on a blackboard. Think about how your heart beats faster when danger threatens or the many changes of sexual arousal that occur with fantasy or in anticipation of a romantic encounter.

There are some headache disturbances that, according to our *current* knowledge, appear not to be based on disturbances of the brain or nervous system. These disorders, according to our *current* knowledge, appear to have no biological cause. The term *psychogenic*—having its genesis in the mind—is used to describe such disorders. This term has been imprecisely used and also misused. I use it here to refer to headache conditions that seem not to be associated with any known biological pain-producing mechanism, although the body's biological responses to anxiety may be present. In these disorders, "pain" is considered to represent the predominant expression of a psychiatric disorder.

The Conversion Headache

In traditional psychological and psychiatric terms, certain patients will experience headaches as a consequence of internal psychological and psychiatric distress or conflict. In such instances, the physical pain of headache is thought to represent a conversion or transfer from psychological disturbance to a physical one.

Some authorities suggest that this condition may begin between ages 20 and 40 and that it is more common in women than in men. Many individuals thought to have this condition have features of immature personalities, including excessive dependency needs. The pain itself does not have any particular quality except that appropriate treatment does not bring relief. The patient may describe the pain in overly dramatic terms. The pain seems to have an overwhelming impact on the patient's life, to an extent greater than seems reasonable. Overuse of painkillers, recruitment of other family members into the search for help, and other unusual features may also be present.

Careful evaluation of patients with this condition will often identify serious and important psychological distress earlier in life or taking place currently. Sexual conflict, problems with morality, or other important considerations are frequently found.

Other Headaches Caused by Psychological Distress

Of course, many types of headaches besides conversion headaches have been ascribed to psychiatric causes. Anxiety, depression, and even psychotic delusion have all been associated with headaches which seem to improve when the primary psychiatric disturbance is ameliorated with treatment.

The treatment of headaches caused primarily by psychiatric illness is, of course, to confront the mental health problem directly. The use of certain medications, psychotherapy, and family interventions are all worthwhile and at times critical.

Changing Concepts of Disease, Brain, and Mind

Before leaving this subject, though, it is important to emphasize certain important historical considerations. First, our concept of mental health has changed over time as we begin to understand more completely the biological factors of the brain and its chemistry. Many psychiatric conditions of the past have now been determined to have been caused by disturbances of brain biology. Among these are manic-depressive disease, schizophrenia, and certain forms of depression. Recent work on brain endorphins and the biogenic neurotransmitters may open new frontiers in our understanding of the relationship between mind and brain, particularly as they relate to pain. It is possible that certain dysfunctions of the brain cause both painful events and psychiatric disturbances, the correction of which brings relief of both symptom groups.

The term hysteria was initially used to describe a condition thought to be the result of a "wandering" throughout the body of the woman's uterus (*hystera*). It was thought that the symptom of hysteria resulted in part from the location in which the wandering uterus sought refuge. It was the belief at the time that the uterus wandered from its original location in search of water or some nutrient. Attempts to control hysteria included placing various substances within the vagina in an attempt to attract the uterus back to its normal location.

We have, of course, come a long way since that time, and our concepts regarding the brain and mind have changed dramatically. There is little doubt that some people experience headache and other symptoms as a direct consequence of psychiatric and psychodynamic disturbances. It is also true that many conditions once originally thought to be the result of primary psychiatric disease have turned out to be caused by neurological disease. We must continue to be open-minded, with flexibility and tolerance for these concepts and our limited knowledge of how the brain and mind work.

13

Headaches That Occur
After Trauma

Trauma means injury, and *posttraumatic* means after an injury. In as many as 50% of cases of head injury, one or more headache patterns develop and persist after the injury itself has healed. The headache is often accompanied by a constellation of other symptoms that are remarkably consistent from patient to patient. This symptom pattern is called *posttraumatic* or *postconcussion syndrome*. I prefer the term posttraumatic, since concussion involves loss of consciousness, and this syndrome may occur even though no loss of consciousness accompanied the injury.

This chapter discusses both posttraumatic headaches and the posttraumatic syndrome of which headache is usually a component. In most patients who experience persistent, recurring symptoms, there are no *obvious* abnormalities within the skull (the cranium) to explain the symptoms. Recent studies suggest that subtle biological abnormalities of the brain are nevertheless present.

Posttraumatic Headache

The incidence of posttraumatic headache varies from 33% to 80%. The headache may take one or more of several forms. Considerable overlap between forms exists, and mixed signs and symptoms are common.

Perhaps the most frequently encountered posttraumatic headache bears striking similarity to typical muscle contraction headaches, and is characterized by constant, nonthrobbing, generalized discomfort. Although it may be confined to one side, both sides are usually affected. The pain is frequently present upon awakening. The discomfort generally extends from the base of the skull to the forehead and, for the most part, cannot be clinically distinguished from muscle contraction headache unassociated with trauma.

A second posttraumatic headache pattern resembles episodic migraine. It is often accompanied by classic migraine features.

Another posttraumatic headache form is characterized by localized discomfort and tenderness to touch. It may have a jabbing, stabbing quality. Throbbing can occur. The pain may be periodic or continuous, with sudden attacks of intense pain. Light pressure such as from a pillow or hat can precipitate an attack of intense pain. This headache form may be related to localized blood vessel and/or nerve injury.

Most posttraumatic headaches resemble the typical mixed headache (see Chapter 10), with coexisting vascular and muscular-like elements. Distinctive patterns like those described above may be superimposed.

The Posttraumatic Syndrome

In addition to headache, minor or more severe head and neck trauma can bring about the development of a set of characteristic symptoms, with striking consistency from patient to patient, but varying greatly in intensity and extent to which they cause disability. This syndrome appears to bear little consistent relationship to the degree of trauma or presence or absence of such features as amnesia, loss of consciousness, blood in the cerebrospinal fluid (CSF), presence of fracture, or other identifiable abnormality. The most commonly reported symptoms include headache, true vertigo or simple dizziness, and personality disturbances including mood changes, most notably depression and anxiety. Impairment of memory and reduced attention span, ringing in the ears (tinnitus), insomnia, and easy fatigability and reduced motivation are also common, as are decreased libido and loss of sexual interest, blurred vision, and alcohol intolerance. In addition, minor neurological findings have been reported. Fainting is described in about 10% of cases and usually accompanies vertigo. The signs and symptoms of posttraumatic syndrome usually develop within 24 to 48 hours after trauma, although they may be somewhat delayed in onset. The dizziness, vertigo, and headaches are typically aggravated by exertion.

Posttraumatic symptoms in children may be identical or may vary from those seen in adults. Hyperactivity, reduced attention span, anger outburst, and bedwetting can represent the main features. When present, headache may not be the predominant symptom.

Causes of Posttraumatic Syndrome

The exact cause of this syndrome is not well understood. There is growing recognition that during trauma, even that associated with whiplash and minor head impact, the contents of the skull (brain) may encounter significant assault. During life, the brain has the consistency of firm Jello, and when the skull is traumatized by impact or rapid jolting, the brain appears to be injured either by coming into direct contact with the skull in the forward and then in the reverse direction, or by energy forces that are absorbed within the brain substance.

Research into this area suggests that even if there is no crushing injury to the brain, the bruising phenomenon or the absorption of energy forces is sufficient to damage brain cells, leading to several possible results. Among these are reduction in neural (nerve) connections and thus in communication between brain parts, impairment of the ability of nerve cells to respond to neurotransmitters, or failure to produce adequate neurotransmittors. As a result, during the days following injury (sometimes even minor ones) individuals report a growing reduction in their ability to concentrate, remember, think through problems, and carry on what would otherwise seem to be everyday tasks. Personality change, growing depression, and a variety of other symptoms are noted.

With respect to the headache itself, as the head comes into contact with an immovable object such as a windshield, or simply is thrust back and forth as in "whiplash," the connection between the neck and head (occipitocervical junction) undergoes significant strain. The muscles, tendons, nerves, and other tissues appear vulnerable to a variety of injuries. Tenderness, stiffness of muscles, and generalized headaches are frequently encountered. Direct trauma to the scalp will not only cause injury to the nerves in the scalp but also an impairment of the blood vessels' ability to constrict and dilate properly.

Moreover, the inner ear mechanism is frequently damaged by this type of injury, disturbing the delicate structures within the bones that house the head's "gyroscope" (the middle ear). The brain can receive abnormal signals when the head is in certain postures, resulting in the sensation of spinning and dizziness, often to the extent that individuals feel as though they are going to fall over or actually do.

Though the symptoms following this type of injury are often dramatic, they are difficult to identify with routine diagnostic techniques. Thus, the patient who has experienced an important change in the ability to function may not demonstrate abnormalities on diagnostic testing. This has led to a serious confusion and disagreement over the legitimacy of this problem.

Because many patients who are injured pursue, for a variety of reasons, legal recourse, many believe that the prolonged symptoms following head injury are in part related to ulterior motives related to litigation and compensation. Although psychological, compensation, and legal issues are unquestionably important to some who suffer these conditions, an increasing body of physicians studying this problem have come to support the legitimacy of most patients with this syndrome.

Of the tests that are likely to identify any existing abnormality, neuropsychological testing appears to be the most valid. During this test, which may last for several hours to all day, the individual is put through a series of mental tasks, puzzles, and maneuvers to test various parts of the brain, how it processes information, and the ability to think through complex tasks. To experienced neuropsychologists, these tests are able to demonstrate abnormalities that are otherwise not definable by standard neurological testing such as CT scans, EEGs, and others. Special EEGs and an electrical study called brain stem evoked responses (BSER) sometimes demonstrate abnormalities as well.

Psychological and Legal Considerations

Anxiety and depression are common in patients with posttraumatic syndrome, but their presence does not mean that their complaints are not legitimate. Preexisting personality and psychological vulnerability may predispose some injured people to more severe emotional reactions to injury and related events. Cynicism of physicians toward patients suffering from posttraumatic symptoms, particularly people in whom psychological disturbances are obvious, may contribute to the perpetuation of symptoms, including hopeless and helpless attitudes. Insensitivity and prejudice deprives the already disturbed person the authoritative explanation and reassurance from their physicians that people need. Sensitivity, reassurance, and warmth are vital in situations where fear, impaired mental function, and uncertainty exist. The challenge is, of course, to distinguish the psychologically or intellectually impaired patient whose symptoms were induced or aggravated by trauma from those in whom the persistence of symptoms is prompted by compensation motives, revenge, or primary and unrelated psychiatric disturbances.

Legal settlement does not necessarily bring a termination of symptoms or a return to work. Moreover, headaches, decreased memory, and depression have been known to develop when no litigation is pending.

Athletes' injuries may also lead to posttraumatic symptoms, though these may be of shorter duration. In one study, 60% of concussed football players experienced headache, and 54% complained of dizziness following head trauma. Seventeen percent lost playing time—80% of whom were unable to participate for at least one week. Those with relatively normal pretrauma personalities also appear vulnerable to posttraumatic symptoms.

Treatment of Posttraumatic Syndrome

The treatment of posttraumatic syndrome and accompanying headaches requires patience, persistence, and understanding. A firm but fair attitude regarding employment matters and an aggressive confrontation of physical and psychological issues are required. Adequate professional time and sufficient reassurance to allay anxiety and fear that a serious brain injury has occurred are essential. Trust and confidence must be established. The physician must engage the patient in a frank discussion of the limits of disability, setting forth early that eventual return to work is expected when appropriate and represents one of the goals of therapy.

Unfortunately, returning to work is complicated by compensation and employment practices, which at times reinforce and encourage disability, the persistence of symptoms, and the prolongation of medical care. Compensation policies that require performance at full capacity as a condition to returning to work make an early, gradual, and protected return most difficult. Patients should be encouraged to attempt part-time or limited activity until full recovery occurs. Unfortunately, a variety of factors including motivational issues of some patients, legal and compensation considerations, and inflexibility by some employers and insurance carriers make this strategy most difficult to carry out.

Recently, I encountered a patient who, on her own initiative, had elected to return to work prior to any reduction of her headaches, which had occurred as a direct consequence of a motor vehicle accident in which she had suffered a concussion. Her return to work was motivated by her own sense of duty and the desire to maintain a constant income for her two children, for whom she was the only support. The insurance company successfully argued that her return to work was evidence that her symptoms were of such little consequence that work was possible, as demonstrated by her work resumption. Subsequent medical bills were therefore not covered by the insurance carrier. Had this patient not returned to work, the same insurers might have argued that she was unmotivated since she was receiving appropriate care to make her better.

Medical Management of Posttrauma Syndrome Various medicines have been used to relieve some of the symptoms of posttraumatic disorder. The combined use of the tricyclic antidepressants, beta blockers, nonsteroidal anti-inflammatory agents (the arthritis drugs), Midrin, ergotamine tartrate, and others can all bring about relief. Their use must be carefully undertaken since too much medicine may aggravate some of the mental changes that have resulted from the injury. Although the symptoms may respond to mild tranquilizers, their use should be restricted. The dizziness that frequently is encountered may respond to specific drugs that calm the inner ear mechanisms. Again, the use of drugs with sedative effects, which many of these have, must be balanced by the recognition that while treating one set of symptoms, one may cause another set of symptoms.

Patients may encounter neuralgic (nerve) pain. This pain is usually "pinpoint" and can be aggravated by pressure with the index finger. Local injections of anesthetic agents (freezing agents) can sometimes help diagnose and treat the condition.

Nerve blocks, or injection of local anesthetic to the area of tenderness around the nerve, can be very helpful for pain in the back of the head (the occipital-cervical junction) and anywhere along the course of a nerve that has been injured. Surgical intervention is sometimes employed to relieve nerve damage and subsequent pain.

Nonmedical Therapy Head trauma is frequently accompanied by neck injury. Thus, heat and massage, ultrasound, traction, and other forms of physical therapy together with support collars and a cervical pillow can be helpful.

Biofeedback and stress management techniques can give the individual with head injury some personal control over the pain and is strongly recommended. Use of electrical devices called transneural stimulators (TENS units) can sometimes provide excellent control over pain and tenderness about the head and neck.

Psychological intervention is quite important. Most individuals who have been injured demonstrated one or more of a variety of psychological consequences that may touch not only the patient but also the patient's family. Many times individuals with head trauma, after receiving initial support and sympathy from caring family members, eventually find themselves rejected as cynicism toward their prolonged symptoms grows. They become burdensome to family members, who begin to doubt the legitimacy of their complaints and symptoms.

Prognosis

It may take many years to recover from this type of injury. Many patients seeking specialists' care experience a protracted course of discomfort from months to years. This does not appear to be directly related to whether litigation issues are present.

We recommend that patients who have had injuries make an attempt to gradually return to normal function, beginning with tasks around the house and progressing to more complicated and paced undertakings. Rehabilitation, vocational training, and a variety of other interventions are necessary. Attempts to work with employers to allow graduated and paced return to full employment is worthwhile, although many employers maintain an "all or none" position.

A complicated problem is one that involves reimbursement and compensation for injury. Because of the complexities of current compensation rules, many patients appear to make more money while sick than while well and working. This is a serious problem because it takes away the normal motivation for returning to work. The solution to this problem will require a coordinated and committed effort between physicians, patients, employers, legislators, and the insurance industry. At this point, little has been done to address this problem.

Summing Up

The available evidence suggests that head and neck trauma, even when ostensibly mild, can produce a constellation of symptoms which may include headache alone, or headache in conjunction with several other disturbances, including mental and mood changes, dizziness and vertigo, insomnia, fatigue, altered motivation and attention span, and a decrease in sexual interest, among others. The consistency of symptoms from one person to another, and the corroborating yet preliminary studies suggesting impairments that could explain the symptoms, cannot be overlooked. Certain pretrauma personality and/or biological factors could serve to predispose an individual to more dramatic reactions of both mind and body to injury or assault than otherwise obvious.

The brain possesses an extraordinary network of sensory organs to judge and respond to the environment and its own function. Perhaps it should not be surprising that this intricate and delicate network possesses a degree of sensitivity and vulnerability to the extent that even mild disturbances or interruption of normal function can result in many of the symptoms and characteristic features of the posttraumatic syndrome. That individuals with preexisting anxiety and emotional vulnerability seem more predisposed to this syndrome can perhaps best be explained by greater attention and concern, or even fixation, by these persons to sensory information or distress, and an excessive biological responsiveness than would otherwise seem natural.

Once symptoms are present, many factors contribute to their worsening, including cynicism regarding the legitimacy of the complaint, neglect of the accompanying anxiety and fear, and the absence of supportive concern generally afforded other illnesses. Headache, dizziness, and decreased mental function should be expected sequels of head trauma and should arouse suspicion only when unduly prolonged or intense, or associated with greater disability than reasonable.

Most people with this syndrome will improve in time. A

supportive, trusting, and well-structured therapeutic program, emphasizing rehabilitation, medical and psychological assessment and management, and reasonable expectations clearly provides the best treatment approach.

14

Additional Conditions
That Cause Headaches

This chapter describes a variety of headache conditions not easily classified under the general category of migraine, muscle contraction, or cluster headache. Many of these headache conditions are related to particular systemic or localized disease processes, in which headache is the first or most prominent symptom. It is possible, in fact likely, that individuals experiencing some of these disorders also suffer from well-recognized chronic headache syndromes, or are at least predisposed to them. Awareness of these headache-producing conditions serves once again to emphasize that headache is a universal symptom and that in the assessment of the complaint of headache it is essential that all major body systems be considered.

Infection

Infection, localized or generalized, may produce headache. The mechanism by which headache occurs is not well understood. It is assumed that in the case of fever-producing conditions, the fever exerts an expanding effect on blood vessels. Localized infection about the head or neck may cause inflammation, swelling, and pressure on sensitive tissue. Meningitis produces headache presumably via involvement of pain-sensitive tissue. In generalized infection, the presence of various toxic substances may have a provoking effect.

Headache associated with fever is usually nonspecific. Throbbing and aggravation from changes in position are common. Simple analgesics will reduce fever and often alleviate the headache. Antimigraine drugs such as ergotamine and Midrin may also be useful. However, these medicines constrict the blood vessels. They may exert an excessive constriction in the presence of fever and should be used with great care, if at all.

Headache due to specific and localized infectious disorders improves following treatment of the particular condition.

Toxins and Medications

The technological and industrial growth of society has made widespread exposure to a myriad of toxins and noxious vapors common. Among the substances found to a greater or lesser extent in industry, agriculture, and the home are turpentine, carbon tetrachloride, benzine (used in gasoline), and benzene (used in leather processing, motor fuels, glue, paints, and linoleums). Mild exposure may produce only headache, but prolonged or excessive exposure can cause serious medical consequences.

Formaldehyde may also produce headaches. People whose homes have been insulated or constructed with formaldehyde-containing products (particle board) may report the onset of headache. Formaldehyde is a suspected cancer-causing agent in laboratory animals.

Various heavy metals, particularly lead, cause headache. Poisoning may occur from contact with chemicals in lead batteries, dabbing of the tongue with an art brush dipped in lead-containing paint, drinking moonshine whiskey made in lead or lead-soldered tubing, drinking from improperly glazed pottery, or living near busy highways or in close proximity to air or water polluting industries.

Carbon monoxide, an odorless poison, may also cause headache. Working in poorly ventilated autoshops or expressway toll booths, driving on highways for long hours, or breathing air from faulty furnaces can result in headache and other symptoms of carbon monoxide exposure. Heavy cigarette smoking may also be a cause.

Medicines may produce headaches or aggravate existing headache disorders. Among these are some antiseizure drugs and blood pressure–lowering medications. Some drugs that are useful in controlling some headache conditions may also produce headaches. Additional headache-producing agents include nitroglycerin and other blood vessel expanders, amphetamines, diet pills, ephedrine, and asthma medications. Birth control pills may provoke headaches or may aggravate existing migraine.

Constipation

Headache associated with chronic constipation does not have special features. Whether a direct link between constipation and headache exists is open to serious question. When present, the headache is usually described as generalized and sometimes throbbing. It may be accompanied by nausea and lightheadedness. Some people who are depressed and those with nerve-related gastrointestinal problems frequently suffer constipation from either psychological factors or medications used to treat their disorders. The relationship between these states and headaches remains unclear.

The cause of the constipation headache, if such actually exists, is unknown. In addition to the psychological possibilities, absorption of toxic substances from the stool or nervous system reactions to the dilated bowel have been proposed.

Collagen Vascular Diseases

Headaches are frequently reported in patients suffering from collagen vascular disease. This section focuses on those disorders in which headache is particularly common.

Temporal Arteritis Temporal arteritis is a generalized inflammation involving primarily but not exclusively the arteries about the head and neck. The disease affects about four times more women than men and generally begins after the age of 50, but it has been reported in younger people. Headache is the most characteristic symptom of temporal arteritis. However, pain in jaw muscles when chewing, visual disturbances (double vision and blindness), weight loss, fever, night sweats, and hypochromic anemia are usually present to some degree in patients whose disease is advanced.

Although headache is the predominant symptom of temporal arteritis, it may not be present in all cases, particularly early in the course of the syndrome. The headache may affect one side or both, often in the temple region. It is usually described as boring or burning, although sharp, lancinating features have been reported. A characteristic feature of the pain is its in the skin location and associated scalp tenderness. Other features include intensification at night and worsening by exposure to cold. The superficial temporal artery is often tender to touch, and the skin overlying the artery is frequently reddened.

Impairment of vision in one eye or both is the most common serious disturbance of cranial arteritis, occurring in up to 50% of untreated patients. Double vision occurs in about 10% of patients. Temporal arteritis may cause permanent blindness and stroke, therefore early treatment is essential.

Systemic Lupus Erythematosus

Headache may occur in an estimated 45% of patients with systemic lupus erythematosus (SLE). The mechanism of headache is not well understood. The headache associated with SLE may be similar and even indistinguishable from classic migraine, and associated with visual disturbances that are discussed in Chapter 4. Headache may be the first symptom of SLE.

Most authorities agree that antimigraine medication is of little value. Administering cortisone or increasing the dosage usually alleviates headache. This therapy would have to be used as part of a comprehensive treatment program.

The Neuralgias

The term *neuralgia* refers to pain arising primarily from a specific nerve branch. Characteristic features of neuralgic syndromes are jabbing, sudden, repetitive attacks of pain. This section will address four important neuralgias.

Postherpetic Neuralgia Postherpetic neuralgia is an intense neuralgic syndrome following herpes zoster, a viral disease of the nerves commonly known as "shingles." It generally affects the facial nerves, though peripheral nerves or roots in the spine may be involved. It usually occurs in people past middle age.

Although mild discomfort may precede or accompany the skin blister that is characteristic of this disease, more intense nerve pain generally occurs following the acute attack. In patients with herpes zoster, this condition affects up to 30% of those over the age of 40, and 50% over the age of 60. The pain is on one side and is persistent. Patients describe it as burning and searing. Periodic attacks of stabbing pain occur. The discomfort may recede spontaneously after several weeks. However, continuous pain for months and even years is not uncommon, particularly in the elderly.

Associated abnormalities include inflammation and scarring of eye tissue, secondary glaucoma, blindness, numbness, and degeneration of skin tissue. Permanent nerve impairment can occur.

There is no specific treatment for postherpetic neuralgia. Sometimes cortisone treatment during the course of the initial infection, and even nerve blocks during that time, can reduce the likelihood of the prolonged painful condition. Once it does develop, however, certain drugs including antiseizure medicine, as well as several others, have been reported to reduce the pain. Nerve blocks at this time might also be effective.

Trigeminal Neuralgia Trigeminal neuralgia is another condition that affects the nerves of the face. It is also called *tic douloureux*. This condition is an intensely painful disorder that affects more men than women. Its name is derived from that of the trigeminal, or fifth cranial, nerve, one of the major nerves of the facial area.

Trigeminal neuralgia causes periodic brief spasms of sudden, intense pain on one side of the face. These "lightning flashes" of pain may recur repeatedly throughout the day. A characteristic feature of this syndrome is the presence of a "trigger zone" which, when stimulated, will produce the intensely painful spasms. Patients tend to avoid chewing, washing their faces, and brushing their teeth on the affected side. The bouts of pain may persist for months before subsiding spontaneously. Recurrence is common. Trigeminal neuralgia may run in families.

Most cases of trigeminal neuralgia occur in people over 50. A similar syndrome occurs in an estimated 1 to 3% of younger people who have multiple sclerosis. The cause of trigeminal neuralgia is uncertain. One possible cause is compression of the trigeminal nerve by a looping or twisted blood vessel from the brain stem.

Trigeminal neuralgia can be treated with drugs or by surgery. Usually, the physician will try medication first. A combination of drugs is sometimes required.

Glossopharyngeal Neuralgia This condition is similar to trigeminal neuralgia, but the affected region is that of the throat, ear, and neck. This area is supplied by the glossopharyngeal nerve. Trigger zones in the throat area may activate sudden, intense pain when the patient eats, swallows, chews, talks, or yawns. Glossopharyngeal neuralgia is less common than trigeminal neuralgia and is treated similarly. If medication does not relieve the problem, portions of the nerve may be surgically sectioned (cut).

Occipital Neuralgia Occipital neuralgia is a disorder involving the occipital nerves, which run from the neck to the head crossing the junction of the head and neck at the base of the skull. These nerves are frequently injured in traumatic events such as whiplash and other conditions that forcibly drive the head backward on the neck and shoulders. Occipital neuralgia can also occur spontaneously and can be caused by viruses that affect nerves, such as herpes zoster.

The pain can be continuous or periodic, and "trigger zones" occur along the course of the nerve. Pressure behind the ear in the region where the neck and head join can produce pain. Placing the head on a firm object—for example, lying on a mattress without a pillow or against the arm rests of a sofa—can produce the painful attack. Attacks can occur spontaneously as well.

This condition can be treated with medicine, nerve block procedures which numb the nerve with a freezing agent such as a local anesthetic, or surgery. Like other neuralgias, it is sometimes difficult to diagnose and can be associated with muscular and sometimes migraine-like discomfort which overshadow and confuse the features of the neuralgia.

Carotidynia

The term *carotidynia* was first used in 1932 to describe pain in the carotid artery, a major blood vessel running along both sides of the neck. The syndrome of carotidynia is characterized by recurring episodes of throbbing discomfort in the neck and lower jaw. The pain is accompanied by tenderness and swelling. A strong relationship between carotidynia and migraine is presumed. Although 50% of patients with migraine experience carotid tenderness during a migraine attack, it may occur in people who do not have typical migraine.

Carotidynia is found in young, middle, or late age. Repetitive attacks may "cluster" over several days. The pain is typically in the neck. The eye and the jaw are frequently affected also. The discomfort is usually described as throbbing. Each attack lasts from several minutes to hours, and tender swelling around the carotid artery is characteristic.

Carotidynia may be treated symptomatically or preventively, depending on the course of the attacks. Ergotamine tartrate is usually effective for symptomatic relief. Methysergide, beta blockers, and nortriptyline have been found effective for prevention. Steroids may be useful for short-term therapy.

Headaches Associated With Stroke and Stroke-Like Conditions

Headaches can occur in association with stroke (cerebrovascular accident). A headache may precede, coincide with, or follow the stroke. Headaches are very frequently a warning sign for bleeding into or around the brain from a bursting aneurysm or blood vessel. There are no distinguishing features which allow this type of headache to be discerned from other nonspecific forms.

As in all cases of sudden, unexpected pain, a headache may be an alert, signaling significant illness. Proper evaluation should be undertaken by a skilled professional.

Hypertension (High Blood Pressure) High blood pressure can be the cause of headache, but in order to produce headache, the blood pressure must be severely high, much more than it generally is in patients with mild to moderate hypertension. During a headache, the blood pressure may also rise to a higher level than usual, causing confusion about whether the elevated blood pressure is due to the headache or the headache due to the blood pressure.

In most patients who have headache, high blood pressure is not the cause. Nevertheless, high blood pressure should always be treated. Ironically, certain medications that are used to control blood pressure can themselves produce headache. If you are being treated for high blood pressure and are having headaches, tell your doctor.

Headaches Related to Exertion

Sexual Activity Many people complain of headache during or shortly after sexual excitement or exertion during sexual activity. Several headache patterns have been identified. A dull bilateral discomfort can occur during the evolution of sexual excitement and is perhaps related to excessive contraction of neck and head muscles. This headache may be alleviated by relaxation.

Another headache form is characterized by intense, explosive head pain occurring just before or during the moment of orgasm. An increase in blood pressure may be responsible for this headache.

A third headache, occurring during intercourse, has distinctive orthostatic characteristics, meaning that it is related to changes in position. It is worse on standing and partially relieved by reclining.

Headaches during intercourse affect more men than women and usually occur in those who have experienced migraine in the past. Similar headaches have been reported during masturbation.

Although headache during sexual intercourse is most often benign, it may reflect more serious conditions. Blood pressure and pulse rate rise markedly during orgasm. A number of serious illnesses can be made worse by this effect.

Termination of sexual activity at the onset of headache usually brings relief within several minutes to an hour or two. Continued activity causes more prolonged and lingering attacks.

Other Exertional Headaches In addition to sexual exertion, head pain may arise during any form of physical exercise or during sneezing, laughing, or yawning. The location of the exertional headache is variable. Throbbing, sharp, and stabbing pain is described. It may last minutes to hours and frequently occurs in those with preexisting headaches. Gastrointestinal and visual symptoms occasionally accompany the headache. All cases of exertional headache require careful examination.

Headache After "Spinal Tap" (Lumbar Puncture)

Approximately one half of patients who undergo a test called a spinal tap, in which fluid is withdrawn from the spine for testing, experience generalized headache. The pain is characteristically worsened by the upright position and relieved by reclining. The headache may be accompanied by neck stiffness and nausea and vomiting. It usually develops within hours of the test.

The physician can sometimes prevent spinal tap headache by using a small-gauge needle to withdraw the fluid and by having the patient recline for several hours after the test. Even under the best conditions, the headache cannot always be prevented.

The best treatment is to remain in the reclining position for as long as possible, take mild analgesics, drink abundant fluids, and avoid any exertion (exercise) for several days.

Headaches Associated With Brain Tumor

Many patients fear that their headaches are due to brain tumors, but most patients with headaches need not worry that the cause of their headache is a serious disease. Only a small number of people who actually have a brain tumor will have headache as an initial symptom. Most cases of brain tumor begin with symptoms other than pain, such as seizures, paralysis, or progressive visual impairment.

The headache associated with a brain tumor is not characteristic. If it does occur, it may be mild or severe, intermittent, and frequently worsened by exertion or posture change. Nausea and vomiting and sensitivity to light may be present, but these are also very common features of migraine.

Features that should alert a person to the possibility of a tumor include the presence of neurological symptoms (numbness, weakness, seizures, progressive visual disturbance, and others) combined with persistent or intermittent headache. If the condition worsens, the treatment does not relieve the problem, or pain persists in the same area of the head, the physician may consider, and test for, possible brain tumor. Even so, features are frequently present in people without serious disease.

Ice-Pick Pain

Some patients with migraine will experience periodic brief and lightning-like jabs of pain lasting only a second or less. Multiple stabs of pain can occur throughout the day. The condition is harmless but frightening.

Headaches Associated With Disease of the Heart Valves

Recently, researchers have identified the possible association of headache, usually migraine, with a condition of the heart called mitral valve prolapse. This condition results from an improper function of one of the heart valves, and its relationship to migraine is not clear.

Among the symptoms that may occur in mitral valve prolapse are rapid heartbeat, fainting, and dizziness. Certain of the medicines used to treat headache may also be useful for mitral valve prolapse. The diagnosis must first be made by your physician. A heart murmur characterized by a "clicking" sound is characteristic for this condition.

Hypoglycemia (Low Blood Sugar)

Fasting or missing meals can produce headache, and absence of food for five hours or more during wakefulness or thirteen hours including sleep time may provoke headaches even if the blood sugar is normal. This vulnerability may be greater in persons with a family history of migraine or other headache, but the actual cause is unknown. Most people who have headaches when missing meals do not have severe abnormalities of their glucose metabolism (hypoglycemia or diabetes). Individuals who believe that their headaches are caused by missing meals, should make a special effort of eating four to six small meals a day. Excessive "junk food" intake is discouraged, and a moderate intake of complex carbohydrates or moderate amounts of protein are recommended. Recent research has established that eating excessive amounts of protein (meat, eggs, cheese) tends to lead to health problems. The relationship of hypoglycemia to migraine is also discussed in Chapter 5.

Headaches and Vitamins

Several of my patients have experienced a worsening of preexisting headaches as a consequence of taking high doses of vitamin supplements. Reduction of vitamin intake brought relief or improvement. Although little is known about the long-term benefits or hazards of high-dose vitamins, it appears that vitamin A and niacin may aggravate headache disorders.

Vitamin A has been found responsible for producing an illness, including headache, experienced by arctic explorers who ingested large amounts of polar bear liver, which is high in vitamin A. The headache has nonspecific characteristics. It frequently occurs daily, on both sides of the forehead or both temples. Throbbing is sometimes present. The headache begins days following the ingestion of at least 25,000 IUs of vitamin A and will generally resolve slowly after discontinuance.

Short-term excess of vitamin A intake results in gastrointestinal distress, vertigo, and malaise. A swelling of the brain, particularly in children, is associated with excessive vitamin A intake.

Long-term ingestion of excessive vitamin A may cause headache, blurred vision, and double vision, along with liver enlargement, joint pain, baldness, fatigue, changes in skin color or texture, inflammation of nerves (neuritis), and fissuring of the lips.

As already mentioned, B vitamins, particularly niacin, can produce headache as well as a flushing reaction. Patients with a headache tendency who take niacin may experience a throbbing discomfort shortly after ingestion.

Alcohol

Alcohol provokes headaches in several ways. During or shortly after drinking, headache may result from expansion of the blood vessels in the head or from the influence of histamine and tyramine present in many liquors.

A hangover represents a constellation of symptoms developing hours after drinking and is characterized by throbbing headache, sensitivity to light, gastrointestinal distress, malaise, and pallor. The syndrome begins after alcohol has been metabolized and when tissue levels of alcohol are low. The hangover headache is similar to migraine, lasts several hours, and is aggravated, like migraine, by movement, rapid postural change, and straining.

Treatment of the hangover headache has historically been based upon a variety of anecdotal and home remedies. Other therapies include aspirin, fructose, or fat ingested prior to drinking, and antimigraine drugs. Oxygen inhalation can be symptomatically beneficial. Because hypoglycemia and dehydration may be important, fluid replacement with sweetened beverages may provide maximum benefit. Coffee may exert an adverse influence because its diuretic action promotes greater dehydration. Recently, research has shown that certain of the arthritis drugs (the nonsteroidal anti-inflammatory agents) may prevent as well as reverse the hangover headache.

Ice Cream Headache

The development of an intense headache moments after ice cold substances are touched to the roof of the mouth is common. The pain is usually dull and nonthrobbing and may be felt in the top of the head, the eyes, or the temples. Other areas about the head are occasionally mentioned.

The so-called "ice cream headache" occurs in approximately 30% of otherwise headache-free people but in up to 90% of those who have a history of migraine. Ice cream headache can be avoided by avoiding ice cream. If you feel that you cannot do without ice cream, eat it slowly so that your palate will cool gradually instead of receiving a shock of cold.

Marijuana

Several of my patients report that marijuana helps relieve their headaches, while others report an intensification of pain (particularly migraine). Although studies have not clearly helped define the issue, it is possible that the relaxing and blood-vessel expanding properties of marijuana may benefit muscle pain (tension headache). On the other hand, the effects of marijuana on the blood vessels and lungs may aggravate migraine.

Disorders of the Head and Neck

Various conditions of the head and neck may also cause headache; for example, patients often think first of eyestrain when they have recurring headache. Actually, conditions of the head and neck actually cause pain far less than they are given credit for.

Headaches Related to Eye Disease

Headaches caused by disorders of the eyes are far less common than is generally supposed. Certain disorders of the eye can cause headache, however. The most important of these are continuing eye strain, inflammation of various parts of the eye, glaucoma, and certain types of tumors that can grow in or around the eye.

Eye Strain When the eyes are fatigued, the muscles that control eye movement are strained. And, when any kind of muscle is strained, pain is often a result. Pain arising from eye strain will worsen when the eyes are used for long periods and improve when the eyes are rested. Eye strain frequently is related to refraction abnormalities—that is, to changes in the lens of the eyes that require the use of glasses or a change in prescription.

Inflammation Certain types of inflammations may also cause eye or head pain. Fortunately, these disorders are relatively rare. Inflammation of the eyes is accompanied by extreme sensitivity to light, burning, and tearing. The eyes may be reddened and tender, and in certain types of inflammation, blurriness of vision is present.

Glaucoma **Primary angle glaucoma** (narrow angle glaucoma) may produce pain around the eye, forehead, or temple region. Pain arising from this type of glaucoma is often accompanied by reduced vision, halos around bright objects, swelling of various parts of the eye, excessive tearing, and dilation of the pupils. Patients with primary angle glaucoma may experience the sudden onset of acute pain in an eye, nausea and vomiting, and changes in pupillary size. It is important to emphasize that these symptoms may also occur in migraine or cluster headache, and it is not unusual for these two conditions to be confused unless a careful evaluation is undertaken.

Fortunately, primary angle glaucoma is a rare illness, but **chronic simple glaucoma** affects approximately 2% of the population over the age of 40. This, the most common form of glaucoma, is the leading cause of acquired blindness but does not cause headaches.

Headaches Related to Diseases of the Ear, Nose, Throat, and Mouth

The Mouth Various conditions of the ear, nose, throat and mouth are also capable of causing headaches. Among these conditions are diseases of the dental structures including gum disease, cracked teeth, abscesses, and afflictions of the nerves going to the teeth. Conditions such as these can produce mouth pain or headache, since the same nerve goes to both areas and the brain may incorrectly locate the origin of the pain.

The Sinuses Sinus disease is a seriously misunderstood problem, and it is now estimated that over 95% of the people who believe that their headaches come from abnormal nasal sinuses actually have no problems with their sinuses at all. The confusion is widespread, but studies to evaluate the association of headache to problems of the sinuses generally fail to show an association in most instances. Acute infections, obstructions, or allergy can of course give rise to sinus pain and tenderness. The pain is generally intense and often made worse by straining and bending over. Frequently there will be fever, nasal drainage, and tearing.

It is important to emphasize that most patients with pain in the sinus area—around an eye, forehead, or temple—do not have sinus disease. Migraine and cluster headache can both cause pressure in these areas, a sense of stuffiness, and even tearing or nasal drainage. Many of the sinus headache medications can help relieve all kinds of headache because they contain mild decongestants, which have a beneficial effect on migraine, and also contain painkillers, which tend to cover up the pain. That a medication designed for sinus disease helps a person's headache, does not prove that sinus headache was present.

Tumors of the throat, nose, and back portions of the nasal cavity can also manifest themselves.

Headaches Related to Disorders of the Jaw

During the past several years there has been increasing interest in the jaw as a cause of headache. Various terms including **temporomandibular joint (TMJ) dysfunction and myofacial pain-dysfunction syndrome (MPD)** have made their way into discussions about headaches. Currently, dental and medical practitioners are involved in considerable controversy about the importance of these conditions as a cause of headache. It is generally agreed that most patients with *serious* and *significant* disturbances of the jaw can experience pain or an aggravation of existing headaches as a result. However, many experienced professionals who specialize in headache treatment believe that the relationship between mild or moderate jaw problems and headache is greatly overstated and overtreated.

I believe that the relationship of jaw disease to chronic and recurring headache has been seriously exaggerated, and many patients who have undergone extensive treatment for their jaws in pursuit of headache control have found themselves disappointed and their condition sometimes worsened. This is not to say that headache or an aggravation of existing headache problems cannot occur as a result of legitimate and confirmed advanced cases of jaw dysfunction. But this is a diagnosis that should come only after careful consideration and more than one opinion.

The primary symptoms of major jaw disease include significant muscle tenderness (the muscles within the mouth and also around the jaw), obvious limitation of normal jaw motion, and marked pain in the joint of the jaw, which is located just in front of the ear canal. The presence of a clicking sound when chewing does not necessarily indicate a serious jaw problem, nor should this condition be assumed to be related to headaches if they are present.

Keep in mind that headache is a common ailment, and so is mild jaw dysfunction. That a person's headache is related to the jaw must be a conclusion that comes after diligent consideration by a variety of professionals of different training and orientation.

Disorders of the Neck

As is the case with the eyes, jaw, and sinuses, the assumption that diseases of the neck are the cause of headaches is seriously overstated. While it is true that serious and important disturbances of the neck can produce headache, it is likewise true that most cases of mild or moderate arthritis in the neck do not cause headache. Significant compression of nerves, herniated disks, *serious* dislocations of the vertebrae (subluxations), and other afflictions of the neck can of course produce pain with resulting headache. However, most patients over the age of 30 have x-ray changes showing neck arthritis, yet most of these individuals do not suffer from headache.

The simple fact that the neck hurts does not necessarily mean that there is something wrong with it. There are many complicated explanations of why the neck may hurt in the absence of disease of the neck. Like all things related to biology, headache and neckache are complicated problems, and simple explanations and solutions are rarely valid.

Headaches and Allergies

The association between headache and allergies is a complicated one. Currently, medical science has not found a direct association between headaches and allergic problems. It is true that some people with allergy to certain foods and other substances can develop a headache or aggravation of existing headache as a consequence, but for most people with chronic recurring headache, allergy is not the cause. It is always wise to consider allergic conditions as a possible provoking influence for headache, but extensive allergy testing in most patients with headaches is not rewarding in terms of finding a meaningful answer.

Sleep and Headache: Sleep Apnea

Many people have headaches when they awaken. Many of the headache disorders already discussed in this book, such as migraine, tension headache, and cluster headache, can be aggravated or brought about by sleeping. Awakening with headache is very common in patients with cluster headaches.

Recently, however, with increasing research it has become clear that some patients who breathe improperly during the night have a condition that has come to be known as *sleep apnea*. This disorder may be caused by disturbances in the brain or may occur if the tonsils or adenoids or some kind of throat swelling blocks the airway. The symptoms of sleep apnea are related to impairment of oxygen intake during the night. People with this disorder will have long pauses during which they do not breathe and then will gasp for air and continue breathing for a while until another pause occurs. During these long pauses, the brain is starved for oxygen, and over time this can have significant and even deadly implications.

Morning headache is sometimes a warning sign of sleep apnea, although it is so common in patients without the condition that it frequently fails to serve as a warning. Patients who snore loudly, have long pauses in breathing, or have other types of major sleep disturbances should be evaluated for this condition. Certain types of medicines and sometimes surgical procedures are useful in correcting this problem.

Summing Up

This chapter has addressed many conditions that can be associated with headache. This information should serve to underline the point that headache can be a warning sign and cannot be taken for granted. Over 300 conditions can cause headache. Fortunately, most of them are innocent and benign, but some are not. Responsible and experienced medical evaluation is essential if we are to benefit from the lessons that modern medical research teaches us.

15

Relaxation Therapy and Biofeedback in Headache Management

Alvin E. Lake III, Ph.D.

Many people with frequent and severe headaches have been told time and time again that if they would only relax, their headache problem would disappear. They may have heard this message from family members, friends, acquaintances, employers, colleagues, and doctors or other health professionals. Although some headache sufferers are eager to explore different methods of relaxation training, others are understandably resentful and frustrated by what they perceive as constant harping on a theme they see as irrelevant to their personal situation. Some of our patients tell us that they have felt dismissed, misunderstood, blamed for their headaches, angry at the doctor or themselves, and left with little direction when this theme was raised. Consequently, we have found that any discussion of relaxation and related therapies such as biofeedback should be handled with sensitivity to the patient's past experiences, and with a clear explanation of what deep relaxation is, why it should be helpful, how best to make use of it, and what to expect.

What Is Deep Relaxation?

Deep relaxation is a learnable skill like riding a bicycle. Some people learn this skill more quickly than others. Anyone willing to make the effort and to continue practice can learn to relax well enough to receive some benefit from it, although the amount of benefit will vary from person to person.

Deep relaxation involves muscle relaxation throughout the head, neck, and body, and dilation of blood vessels in the hands and feet, leading to a sense of warmth in the fingers and toes. Research has also found a significant increase in blood flow to some areas of the brain, as well as a reduction in blood flow through facial arteries that may be swollen during a migraine attack. These changes in blood flow are primarily caused by a decrease in the amount of catecholamines (the components of adrenaline) secreted by nerve cells and circulating through the bloodstream. In addition, there is a shift of blood flow from large muscles to the digestive organs, with an increase in stomach motility and salivation. There may be some watering of the eyes. A person with perspiring hands may notice his or her palms becoming less moist as well as a general decrease in perspiration.

Why Should Relaxation Help?

Muscle tension in the head and neck area contributes to both migraine and muscle contraction headaches, although the nature of this contribution is complex. Some people have headaches that are consistently more intense when their facial muscles are more contracted, although this finding does not hold for all. Researchers have shown that some headache patients may be abnormally sensitive to muscle contraction, developing headaches in response to even brief periods of muscle tension whereas the person who is not headache prone will not. Holding muscle tension (bracing) for a long period of time leads to pain because the contracted muscles create toxic byproducts such as lactic acid and reduce blood flow and oxygen to the affected area. Consequently, the ability to identify the presence of muscle tension before pain develops and to relax the affected muscles would appear to be helpful in preventing or modifying pain.

Chronic muscle tension can be maintained by a reflex between the muscle fibers and the spinal cord. This reflex, involving the muscle spindle system, helps maintain muscle tone. In order to relax the muscle below the resting level of muscle tone, nerve cells originating in a conscious part of the brain called the parietal cortex must be involved. Once a person understands the concept of heavy and loose musculature, focused conscious attention can allow the muscles to relax. Repeated practice of muscle relaxation may then reset the muscle spindle reflex and maintain a lower level of muscle tone.

Both migraine and muscle contraction headaches involve some difficulties with blood flow. In muscle contraction headache, there is a reduction in blood flow to the affected area. In migraine, blood flow through certain blood vessels becomes increasingly variable up to three days before the headache develops. During the throbbing period of pain, the blood vessels in a focused area expand and swell. There is also some recent evidence of a decrease in blood flow to some areas of the brain preceding and during migraine. Consequently, the effect of deep relaxation on stabilizing blood flow, increasing blood flow through constricted vessels, and increasing blood flow to the brain would be expected to have some beneficial effect in preventing this type of headache.

Relaxation might also be expected to help for other reasons including its use as a distraction from pain, its potential to reduce emotional reactions varying from frustration and anger to panic and depression which are often part of the experience of severe or chronic pain, and its potential to help the headache sufferer see him- or herself as less of a victim of the body's whims and as more of a pilot in control of at least some of the body's responses.

How Does One Develop a Relaxation Response?

There are many methods of developing a relaxation response. In 1929, Dr. Edmund Jacobson first outlined a detailed method for the **progressive relaxation** of the skeletal muscles. He also described the successful treatment of four cases of muscle contraction headache. Dr. Jacobson's method involved focusing attention on different muscle groups in order to consciously relax them. More recently, clinicians and researchers have shortened the method, using a cycle of first tensing and then releasing isolated muscle groups while thinking of "continuing to let go farther and farther."

An alternative to progressive relaxation, known as **autogenic**

training, was developed independently in the 1920s by Dr. Johannes Schultz, a Viennese neuropsychiatrist. This approach relied on the silent repetition of thoughts such as "my legs are heavy" or "my hands are warm." Instead of telling the patient to consciously produce a relaxation effect, Schultz encouraged use of these thoughts as if they were "keys" that would automatically unlock the desired effect. Dr. Elmer Green and his wife, Alyce, expanded these phrases to include a shift in attention from the heaviness in the feet to smoothness in the muscles of the face and neck, warmth in the hands, and a quiet mind.

Other methods may involve attention to abdominal breathing and extended periods of 5 to 10 seconds for each inhalation and exhalation, the use of positive imagery such as a trip to a beach, and methods of shifting attention relatively quickly from one area of the body or thought to another, as a means of quieting the background stream of consciousness. Whatever the method, a mental attitude of passive attention is more effective than competitive striving to achieve the effect.

What Is Biofeedback?

The term *biofeedback,* or biological feedback, refers to a method of bringing immediate information about internal physiological processes into conscious awareness. Typically, feedback consists of an oscillating tone, the movement or deflection of a meter, a digital readout, colored light, or a number of lights illuminated in a column. Feedback may also be limited to praise or comments from a therapist observing the electronic equipment.

The goal of biofeedback training is for the person to learn control over muscle tension and blood flow. Obviously, learning to relax the forehead and neck or to increase blood flow through the hands while receiving feedback in a therapists's office is not enough. The person must eventually produce these changes without feedback and when needed during the course of daily life. Consequently, assessment of the person's response to discussion of relevant real-life situations and stressors, as well as typical postures and movements, is a frequent part of biofeedback treatment.

Historical interest in relaxation and meditative techniques can be traced back over hundreds if not thousands of years. Biofeedback, on the other hand, is a relatively recent phenomenon. Although the first reports of using biofeedback for muscle relaxation came from Dr. Jacobson in the early 1950s, it was not until 1969 that a clinical instrument for increasing deep muscle relaxation by means of analog information feedback was described. The first reports on using other methods of biofeedback for the management of migraine began to appear in the early 1970s.

Today there are three commonly used methods of biofeedback training for headache:

Electromyographic (EMG) Feedback In this form of biofeedback, surface electrodes are placed on the skin over specific muscle areas. Typically, three electrodes are placed on the forehead, one over the frontalis muscle above each eye, with a ground electrode half-way between. Other common placements include: 1) the back of the neck or shoulder area over the trapezius muscle, which lies directly under the skin from near the bottom of the skull to across the shoulder and part of the upper back; 2) the cheek area over the masseter muscle which controls biting; and 3) above and slightly in front of the ear in the hairline over the temporalis, another major muscle controlling the jaw. The electrical force generated during muscle tension is measured in microvolts (millionths of a volt). The biofeedback equipment amplifies this extremely low signal while making sure that other sources of electrical energy, such as 60 cycle current from electrical lines, do not affect the signal.

Finger Temperature (Thermal) Feedback This commonly used type of biofeedback involves recording finger temperature with a thermistor, a device that transforms heat into electrical energy so that it can be metered. It is attached to the skin with porous paper tape so that heat is not trapped between the tape and the skin to artificially increase temperature. The thermistor is commonly placed on the pad of one finger, although other sites such as the back of the finger are quite acceptable. It is common for one hand to be somewhat warmer than the other, so consistent use of the same recording site for one individual is important for comparative purposes. As noted in the above discussion of relaxation, finger temperature will increase as blood flow increases to the hands during relaxation. Finger temperature can vary from room temperature (about 72 degrees Fahrenheit) to as high as 95 or 96 degrees. Some heat is lost through the skin, so finger temperature will never quite reach the normal blood temperature of 98.6 degrees. If the blood vessels are fully dilated, finger temperature will reach 95 degrees or more. As a general rule, people with finger temperatures below 80 degrees would feel cold. The low to mid 80's would feel cool, the low 90's would feel warm, and the mid 90-degree range would feel comfortably hot.

Extracranial Blood Volume Pulse Feedback A third form of biofeedback for migraine and other vascular headaches relies on recording the relative volume of blood flowing through the extracranial artery and surrounding tissue over or near the site of pain in the head. A photoplethysmograph, consisting of a light emitting diode and photoelectric cell, is placed over a small surface area of skin. As the heart pumps blood through the artery, the skin becomes more opaque during each pulse, and the photodetector records a reduction in the intensity of reflected light. In this way, the photophlethysmograph can give information on the relative volume of blood from one pulse to another. By watching a feedback display such as a series of lights reflecting the relative amount of blood averaged over several heartbeats, the person can attempt to constrict the swollen or dilated blood vessel that is part of the cause of head pain. This technique shows considerable promise in the treatment of migraine but has primarily been used in research settings and is rarely found in clinical practice at this time.

How Effective Is Relaxation and Biofeedback Therapy?

Overall Effectiveness Although no treatment is universally effective for all people with headaches, both relaxation therapy alone and biofeedback training are of significant benefit for many. Dr. Edward Blanchard and his colleagues found that the average percentage of headache improvement from studies for people with migraine was 65% for those treated with a combination of thermal biofeedback and autogenic training, 52% for thermal biofeedback alone, and 53% for relaxation training alone. In contrast, placebo medication (inactive "medicine") led to only 17% improvement. For those with muscle contraction headache, the average percentage improvement from forehead EMG biofeedback alone was 61%. The rate was 59% for the combination of EMG biofeedback and relaxation training and 59% for relaxation training alone. In contrast, placebo medication and "psychological placebo" (inactive psychological "treatment" such as incorrect feedback) led to average improvements of only 35% each. Simply asking participants to keep headache records without any additional treatment actually led, on the average, to a slight increase in headache activity. These results on the whole held up over follow-up periods of varying lengths. The average improvement for biofeedback and relaxation treatments at follow-up ranged from 57 to 70%. Studies of extracranial blood volume pulse feedback have shown improvement rates from 56 to 71%.

Although these results would suggest that biofeedback has few advantages over relaxation therapy, Dr. Blanchard and his colleagues later showed that the addition of biofeedback training can lead to a significant improvement for people who received little benefit from relaxation training alone. For example, 78% of headache sufferers with mixed migraine/muscle contraction headaches who were not helped by progressive relaxation training were helped at least somewhat by thermal biofeedback. For migraine, 43% of the relaxation "failures" showed at least a 50% improvement after thermal biofeedback training. Similar results were reported for muscle contraction headache patients who received EMG biofeedback after failing to respond to relaxation training, with 47% of the relaxation "failures" reducing headache by at least 50% after a course of EMG biofeedback.

Cluster headache has been much more difficult to relieve with relaxation and biofeedback procedures, although there are a few published cases showing significant improvement for a small number of individuals with thermal or extracranial blood volume pulse biofeedback. Published studies suggest that roughly one out of four people with cluster headaches may derive some benefit.

We have found that some cluster headache sufferers do get a great deal of help from relaxation techniques. Those who are helped in some cases practiced for months or years before developing a reasonable ability to relax during periods of excruciating pain. Some had previously resorted to banging their heads against walls as a method of distraction during the peak of a cluster headache attack. These patients report that their efforts at learning alternative relaxation and distraction techniques have been worthwhile.

At this time there is very little published literature on the use of relaxation and biofeedback therapy with posttraumatic head pain. However, our clinical experience and the results of those studies that are available support the idea that many patients willing to practice these procedures can derive meaningful benefit.

Relieving Acute Pain Biofeedback is both a method of relieving acute pain and preventing headache. To better understand the effectiveness of biofeedback skills in these two aspects of headache control, Jeff Pingel and I completed a follow-up study of 154 randomly selected patients who had completed biofeedback training at our center up to four years previously. The majority of these patients (69%) reported experiencing both migraine and muscle contraction pain, and 67% of this group reported daily pain before beginning treatment, with one-third experiencing constant headache. At the time of follow-up, 56% of the combined migraine/muscle contraction headache patients reported at least a 50% improvement. Improvement was maintained over time, with 57% of those who completed treatment two to four years previously continuing to report at least 50% overall improvement.

The impact of biofeedback training on managing acute

pain for these patients is depicted in Table 5. As shown, 95% reported some ability to remain calm during the headache. In contrast, people were significantly less likely to stop an existing headache, with only one-half reporting any success in stopping migraine. Although not shown in this table, only 8% said they could consistently stop migraine headaches with biofeedback, with 15% noting a consistent ability to stop muscle contraction pain. Given these findings, we have encouraged our patients to think of *relaxing despite the pain*, rather than focusing on reducing the pain. This shift in focus has helped many people control their emotional response to the headache while avoiding frustration if the technique does not reduce the intensity of pain itself.

TABLE 5

Percentage of Mixed Headache Patients Reporting Some Ability to Control Headache With Biofeedback Skills

Type of Control	Type of Headache	
	Migraine	Muscle Contraction
Remain calm	95%	95%
Reduce intensity	81%	92%
Take less pain medication	80%	87%
Reduce duration	73%	89%
Stop headache	49%	68%

Preventing Headaches Table 6 shows the effectiveness of biofeedback for this group in preventing headache. As shown, 80 to 84% reported some ability to prevent headaches previously triggered by stress. In contrast, only about one-third said they could prevent migraine headaches triggered by other factors such as the menstrual cycle, weather changes, and foods. Biofeedback was also significantly more effective in preventing nonstress-related muscle contraction pain than nonstress-related migraine. Other researchers have also found the menstrual migraine to be difficult to control with biofeedback.

TABLE 6

Percentage of Mixed Headache Patients Reporting Some Ability to Prevent Headaches With Biofeedback Skills

Type of Prevention	Type of Headache	
	Migraine	Muscle Contraction
Headaches previously triggered by stress	80%	84%
Headaches previously triggered by other factors	34%	56%

Given the potential of biofeedback, even for some of those with severe pain that does not appear to be stress-related, we routinely encourage all patients in our hospital program to experiment with relaxation techniques during acute pain as well as on a preventive basis at other times. We tell them that although we cannot guarantee results, it makes good sense to seriously experiment with self-management tools such as relaxation in addition to innovative medical treatment.

What Accounts for Headache Improvement With Biofeedback?

Level of Physiological Control Some studies have shown a statistical relationship between the degree of physiological control achieved during training and headache improvement. Specifically, migraine patients who succeed in raising finger temperature to at least 95°F (almost total vessel expansion) and muscle contraction headache sufferers who lower forehead EMG below one microvolt (almost total muscle relaxation in that area) are more likely to show improvement than those with less control. However, many patients who are unable to meet these criteria still report excellent benefits, and some patients who do meet these criteria show no significant improvement. Although important, the level of physiological control shown during training may not be as critical as other factors described below.

Frequency of Relaxation Practice At the beginning of this chapter I highlighted the physiological reasons why relaxation and biofeedback assistance might be of value in headache management. In our follow-up research, Jeff Pingel and I found that daily brief use of relaxation techniques made the most important contribution to overall headache improvement. Sixty-nine percent of those with overall improvement of 50% or better were using brief relaxation techniques daily, in contrast to only 39% of those with less than 50% improvement. These differences are very significant in a statistical and scientific sense. We also found that the majority of our patients (53%) who reported at least a 50% overall improvement continued to practice extended periods of relaxation for 10 minutes or more at a time at least once a week in contrast to only one out of three patients reporting less than a 50% improvement.

It is of some interest that two-thirds (66%) of the mixed headache patients in our study said that either "brief periods of relaxation during the day" or "awareness of thoughts and feelings related to headache" was the most helpful part of biofeedback therapy. Only 7% reported that "regular practice of relaxation for 10 minutes or more at a time" was of most help. We found no relationship between overall improvement and sex, age, frequency of headaches before training, or the years since completing biofeedback.

Belief in Self-Control A positive biofeedback experience can strengthen a person's confidence in his or her ability to control not only hand temperature or muscle tension but headaches as well. In a creative study by Dr. Ken Holroyd and colleagues, tension headache sufferers who were led to believe on the basis of positive feedback that they were very successful in controlling their muscle tension during biofeedback training showed significantly more headache improvement (53%) than those who were led to believe that they were only marginally successful (26%). In this study, the person's belief that he or she could control headaches was a much better predictor of improvement than the actual degree of control over muscle tension. Even people who increased their muscle tension showed good improvement if they were given feedback suggesting a high level of success.

Why should belief make a difference? In my experience, the demonstration that a person is able to modify physiological processes that he or she previously believed to be involuntary, such as hand temperature, has an immediate and dramatic effect on the person's sense of what is possible through self-control. This belief factor may be important in encouraging an individual to pay more attention to his or her body and to use brief relaxation techniques and other biofeedback skills more frequently. It may also encourage more frequent use of stress and pain management techniques that a person has learned in the past but is not using very often now. There is even some recent research showing that people who have been trained to develop increased belief in their ability to control anxiety release significantly less catecholamines into the bloodstream when confronted with a stressor. Catecholamines are the neurotransmitters associated with the so-called fight/flight response. As noted in the discussion at the beginning of this chapter on the physiological basis of relaxation, this reduction in catecholamine level is probably what accounts for the relaxation effect.

What About Biofeedback and Medication?

For some patients, biofeedback can be an alternative to preventive medication. In our follow-up research described above, Jeff Pingel and I found that 64% of the patients using preventive medication said that biofeedback skills helped them reduce the level of preventive medication necessary for headache control, and 37% had eliminated such medication.

For other patients, a combination of biofeedback and medication may be most effective. Several studies have now shown that the combination of biofeedback with drugs such as propranolol (Inderal) or amitriptyline (Elavil or Endep) may be more effective than either medication or biofeedback alone. In our follow-up study, we found that the majority of patients (57%) identified the combination of biofeedback skills and medication as most helpful, and others were evenly divided about which type of treatment they felt was of most help.

However, certain types of medication may need to be discontinued for biofeedback to help. The daily use of pain relievers or vasoconstrictors such as Cafergot will interfere with any other type of treatment including biofeedback by promoting continued "rebound" pain. Also, the frequent use of benzodiazepines (minor tranquilizers such as Valium) can interfere with biofeedback, partly because they detract from the motivation to use biofeedback skills.

Finally, since relaxation and biofeedback involve skill learning and conditioning, several weeks may pass before clear benefits are achieved. The person beginning a program of relaxation or biofeedback therapy should plan to allow at least six weeks of daily relaxation practice before making any judgment of the extent to which treatment is helping. In contrast, medication may work more quickly, with at most a two-week interval between beginning use of a preventive medication and achieving the maximum therapeutic effect at that dosage.

Are There Side Effects from Relaxation and Biofeedback?

Positive Side Effects Most of our patients report positive side effects from biofeedback training. For example, three out of four patients in our follow-up study reported that biofeedback helped them fall asleep or improved overall mood. Also, as noted above, biofeedback training may lead to a greater sense of one's ability to control his or her body, which in itself may be a significant benefit. In fact, one research study reported by Dr. M. Sovak found that people who achieved migraine control with temperature biofeedback also showed a significant improvement in psychological test scores on the Minnesota Multiphasic Personality Inventory (MMPI). In contrast, patients who showed a similar degree of headache improvement following treatment with propranolol (Inderal) did not show similar psychological benefits.

Negative Side Effects In general, relaxation and biofeedback training lead to few if any negative side effects. However, Jeff Pingel and I did find that a minority (20%) of those undergoing our biofeedback program experienced some minor side effects such as drowsiness. A very small minority (5 out of 154 patients) identified side effects they felt were very disturbing, including some distortion in body image such as feeling that their body was growing larger or smaller. It was of some interest for us to find that patients reporting some negative biofeedback side effects were actually more likely to experience a better level of headache improvement. Three of the five patients reporting "very disturbing" side effects noted an overall improvement greater than 75%.

It may be helpful to compare the incidence of biofeedback side effects with medication side effects. In our study, we found that 88% of the patients using preventive medication reported some negative drug effects. Weight gain, drowsiness, fatigue, and dry mouth were each noted by about half of the patients. Approximately 25% of the patients found their medication side effects to be very disturbing, in contrast to only 3% reporting very disturbing biofeedback side effects—a very significant difference. Also, patients continuing to use preventive medication were significantly more likely to report continued negative drug effects in contrast to the short-term nature of most of the negative biofeedback effects.

Is the Benefit Worth the Cost?

In 1986, the total cost for an 8- to 10-session course of biofeedback training was on the order of $600. Some insurance carriers cover some or most of the cost; others do not provide any coverage. Although it may be argued that improvement in quality of life cannot be measured in dollars alone, it is understandable that both insurance companies and the consumer would want to know whether they could expect some offset of future medical costs for their investment. Is the benefit worth the expense?

One recent study by Dr. Edward Blanchard and his colleagues compared the estimated headache-related medical expenses from tax and medical records of biofeedback recipients for the two years prior to treatment to the two years after the completion of training. They found a dramatic change. Estimated expenses for medication, physician's visits, hospital costs, and other nonmedical therapy dropped from an average of $950 per patient before treatment to an average of only $52 per patient after treatment. These figures do not include the cost of the relaxation and biofeedback treatments.

At the time of this writing, there were no other available comprehensive studies of the cost versus benefits of biofeedback, and generalizations from this one study should be made with care. However, the evidence clearly indicates that biofeedback can help dramatically reduce medical costs for some people.

Summing Up

Relaxation and biofeedback are learnable skills that can be useful to many patients in managing problem headaches. Several different types of biofeedback and relaxation procedures have been shown to be effective treatments for migraine and muscle contraction pain. These treatments are less effective for cluster headache, although some people may still benefit. They may also help patients with posttraumatic head pain, although the degree of help has not been well evaluated for this disorder. People who fail to respond to a course of relaxation therapy may still show a significant improvement in headache control with the addition of biofeedback.

Biofeedback can help in relieving acute pain as well as preventing headaches. Most people can learn some ability to remain calm during acute pain, and one out of two report *some* ability to stop migraine. These treatments appear most effective in preventing stress-related headache, although they may help some people prevent headaches triggered by other factors. Improvement has been maintained for several years following treatment.

Headache improvement is related to the continued practice of relaxation, and in particular to the use of brief relaxation techniques on a frequent, daily basis. Biofeedback can also help strengthen a person's belief in his or her ability to control headaches, which may further help account for the benefits. The level of physiological control developed during training may also be important.

Biofeedback therapy can reduce or eliminate the need for medication, although for many the combination of biofeedback and medication may be most effective. On the other hand, the daily use of pain relievers or tranquilizers such as

Valium can interfere with the effectiveness of relaxation and biofeedback.

Most patients report some additional positive benefits from biofeedback training, although a small percentage report negative side effects. There is some evidence that patients reporting negative side effects may also be more likely to report a greater degree of headache improvement than those reporting no negative side effects. Biofeedback-related negative side effects are much less common, less disturbing, and more temporary than negative drug effects.

There is accumulating evidence that biofeedback is a cost-effective treatment that has been shown to lead to a substantial reduction in medical and hospital expenses for some people.

Finally, relaxation and biofeedback have helped make headache therapy a truly cooperative enterprise between the doctor or health professional and patient, where the person takes an active role in his or her own treatment. Instead of the doctor doing something to the patient, the headache sufferer can actively participate in doing something for him- or herself.

16

Cognitive-Behavioral Therapy for Headache

Alvin E. Lake III, Ph.D.

Successful headache therapy often requires some change in a person's behavior. For example, life stress reduction, avoidance of headache triggers such as chocolate or alcohol, and maintaining consistent sleep patterns all rely on behavioral change. Relaxation and biofeedback therapy require use of these skills in daily life. Even drug therapy depends on behavior—the patient's using prescribed medication appropriately.

The term *cognitive-behavior therapy* refers to a specific educational model of teaching headache-relevant coping skills. In this form of treatment, the patient first learns to identify connections between thoughts (cognitions), emotions, behaviors, and pain. The therapist then helps the patient develop alternative thoughts and behaviors that are useful in reducing emotional arousal. After presenting a framework for cognitive-behavioral assessment, this chapter will illustrate how changes in thoughts and behaviors can help reduce the impact of headache on a person's life.

Cognitive-Behavioral Assessment: Antecedents and Consequents

A great deal can be learned from the careful examination of events, situations, thoughts, and behaviors that are associated with an increase in headache. *Antecedents* are events that precede a headache. Antecedents may vary from the time of day to specific foods, bright lights, and confrontations with other people. Antecedents may also include aspects of the person's own thoughts and behaviors, such as self-criticism, self-imposed deadlines, habits of rushing from one task to another, anxiety or worry, sleeping late in the morning, or missing meals. *Consequents* are events that happen as a result of headache. Consequents can be external, such as the ways in which other people treat the person when he or she is in pain. Consequents also involve the person's own thoughts and behaviors, such as self-blame, jaw clenching or muscle contraction in response to pain, a forced period of rest, beginning a mad flurry of activity "before the real headache hits," the use of powerful pain-relieving drugs, the avoidance of unpleasant situations, or the loss of time at work or school.

Case Illustration The chart in Table 8 shows the antecedents and consequents of headaches experienced by a 33-year-old housewife in our practice. This woman had a 13-year history of one-sided headaches with accompanying vascular changes and sensory disturbances.

TABLE 7

A Patient's Cognitive-Behavioral Analysis of Her Headache Episodes

Antecedents (Triggers)	Consequents (Effects)
Kids screaming.	Yell at the kids—"Goddam it you two, shut up!".
Child's constant "How come?"—won't bring one on, but can make it worse.	Say to my daughter "I have a headache," and she gets very quiet. Get mad at myself—get irritated at myself for yelling at the kids—they are little, they don't understand
Husband's work: Long hours —"He's a workaholic. It's a pain to eat dinner between 7:30 and 9:30 at night."	Ask my husband to come home; he did five times since January.
In-laws, when they call. Partiality to one of the kids. Criticism of one child—"She's slow." Criticism of me—"Too bad you don't know how to cook, or I could get you dishes for Christmas." Just hearing my mother-in-law's voice and the top of my head starts to hurt.	Grouchy. Slam the door. Thoughts—"I've got to go to sleep, be able to lie down and have it quiet."

Antecedents (Triggers)	Consequents (Effects)
Mother telling me, "You don't need to go to Ann Arbor for treatment."	Cancel plans—I prefer to cancel than to go and "take somebody's head off."
Thinking of the drive to MHNI my head got tighter and more painful.	Sometimes I don't want to go anyway.
Time pressure.	Got out of going to lunch with husband's secretary.
Loud noises, traffic, TV.	

This analysis revealed several interesting patterns. First, it appeared that her headaches may have unconsciously helped her control her family. She noticed that her child's screaming and constant questioning often aggravated a headache, but that by complaining of head pain she was able to quiet her daughter. Also, she literally described her husband's long hours and late dinners as "a pain." Although she had been unable to make him change his behavior, she had been able to get him out of the office five times during the previous six months in order to come home and take care of her. A second pattern involved her emotional response to certain situations, including criticism from her in-laws and thoughts such as thinking ahead about the drive to the Michigan Headache and Neurological Institute. A third pattern involved anger at herself during a headache, which most likely increased her head pain. Finally, she noted that she had occasionally cancelled plans when "I don't want to go anyway," raising the possibility that her headaches may have helped her avoid some unpleasant activities.

As a result of this assessment, treatment involved a combination of strategies: 1) Instruction in child management skills so that she could develop better methods of calming her children other than raising her voice, slamming doors, and complaining of head pain; 2) some attention to ways she could help improve communication with her husband so that she would not need to rely on headache as a means of "controlling" him; 3) biofeedback-assisted relaxation training with additional rehearsal of using relaxation as a means of coping with criticism, worry, and anger at herself; and 4) focus on learning specific social skills that could make social engagements more rewarding rather than something to be avoided. Further assessment also revealed yearly cycles of depression during the winter months which was treated with medication (lithium).

Five months following the initial assessment this woman reported a 90% improvement in her headache. This improvement was maintained at least until my final contact with her 2 years later. I talked with her husband several months after that, and he also described marked improvement in both his wife's headache and her ability to handle stress. Although it is not possible to identify what parts of the treatment plan were most helpful, this example does illustrate the usefulness of this type of antecedent-consequent analysis in developing a comprehensive and effective treatment plan.

Dealing With Headache-Related Cognitions

Many people with frequent and severe headaches experience intense negative emotional reactions to pain, such as depression; anger at the headache, at themselves, or at other people; or feelings of frustration, helplessness, resentment, disgust, inadequacy, or guilt. These feelings tend to be associated with thoughts such as "When will this end?" "Why does it have to be another headache?" "There's nothing anyone can do." "Am I doing this to myself? I should be in better control." "Other people don't understand." "I can't stand this." "I'm letting my family down." Some people even become upset about being upset, such as becoming angry at themselves for failing to maintain better emotional control.

These feelings and thoughts are understandable reactions to chronic pain and are felt to some extent by most if not all people with frequent and severe headaches. On the other hand, these thoughts and feelings rarely seem beneficial to the person in pain. In some cases, the emotional arousal actually increases headache as if fuel were being poured on a fire. In other cases, the emotional distress does not aggravate the pain but leaves the headache sufferer feeling like an emotional wastebasket. Very few people ever find these feelings helpful to them in reducing pain.

During periods of intense pain, many people find it more helpful to focus on reducing the negative emotions associated with pain and remaining calm despite the pain, rather than focusing on attempting to reduce the pain itself. Successful management of the emotional side of pain can change the entire pain experience, so that what remains is an unpleasant, intense—but much more tolerable—situation. In contrast, focusing only on reducing the sensory component of pain can sometimes lead to further frustration and increased emotional distress.

One useful method of dealing with these negative emotional reactions involves first identifying the specific types of negative thoughts the person experiences during pain, and then developing a written list of alternative coping thoughts for review during periods of intense discomfort.

> Case Illustration. A 37-year-old woman in our practice reported an intense anger and resentment at the beginning of headache episodes. These feelings were associated with a series of negative thoughts, illustrated in Table 8. After creating a detailed and exhaustive list of the negative thinking shown in this table, we constructed together a set of alternative, believable coping responses to correspond with each type of negative thought in the list. At the end of this list she included some positive self-reinforcement ("Good job." "It's hard for me to think these coping thoughts but I tried and at least I made an effort").

TABLE 8

Modification of a Patient's Negative Thoughts
Related to Anger and Resentment
at the Onset of a Headache

Negative Thoughts	Coping Thoughts
I'm not going to be able to control them [my headaches].	• There's no point or value in trying to predict the future course of my headaches.

Negative Thoughts	Coping Thoughts
• Why me? Why do I have these headaches?	• I have a biological predisposition toward headache, just as other people have a predisposition toward diabetes or high blood pressure.
• Are the headaches going to interfere with what I have to do?	• I usually go on and do things anyway. They don't interfere with what I have to do, just my enjoyment is affected. I still enjoy these things, just not as much as if I didn't have a headache.
• I'm stuck with it.	• Don't think about that right now—think about it later.
• What did I do wrong?	• Thinking about what I did or did not do never got me out of a headache. There's no point to it. Maybe I did not do anything wrong anyway. Maybe 100% of my headaches are *not* related to something I did wrong.
• What can I do about it? There's nothing I can do about it. I have no use for them.	• This is an opportunity to try thinking and reacting to it differently. Try it and see what happens. Relax—use your relaxation techniques.
	• Good job. It's hard for me to think these coping thoughts but I tried. At least I made an effort.

Note that the coping thoughts *do not* include "I am not going to get this headache." Although most headache sufferers try this type of wishful thinking at one time or another, it rarely helps much. Too often, it leads to frustration if the headache grows in intensity. Most of our patients find it much more useful to focus on remaining calm despite the headache rather than talking to themselves about the headaches going away.

This patient was a highly educated health professional. At first she said that she thought that writing all this down was rather silly—a mature woman should not need such a list, in her opinion. However, she reluctantly agreed to carry the list with her so that she could experiment with reading the coping thoughts to herself immediately at the onset of headache. At her next session a week later, this woman said, "It took the panic edge off the headache. I really wasn't expecting it to help. I was surprised, I have to say." She continued to find that reading the list of rational thoughts was useful to her and continued to apply it for many months later.

In my experience, people often believe at first that reading or repeating rational coping thoughts will not help them. However, as in this example, people who are willing to experiment with this approach despite their scepticism frequently find that the benefit is well worth the effort. Repetition is also extremely important: Well ingrained negative thoughts do not die easily.

Dealing With Headache-Related Behavior

Although the pain of severe headache is the most pressing concern for almost everyone, the impact of pain on a person's life can be equally distressing. In some cases, a vicious cycle occurs in which the person begins doing less of his or her normal activities either because these activities aggravate headaches or because they seem less enjoyable. If pain continues, a downward spiral can occur, making life less rewarding and increasing the amount of attention devoted to pain. Although pain relief remains a central goal in headache treatment, in some cases it is just as important to help the person return to a more normal life-style despite the continued presence of discomfort. If a person gradually reduces work and leisure pursuits, a worsening depression is almost the inevitable result. If family members begin to take on more and more of the normal responsibilities of the person in pain, the person will begin to see him- or herself as more and more "sick" with a further loss of self-esteem.

A common pattern we have seen too often with some of our younger patients involves a gradual reduction in school attendance, so that when the child first comes for treatment he or she may not be attending school at all. As children become more isolated from classmates, they tend to feel more and more worried about being able to attend school and function if they are still in pain. Understandably, the family becomes more concerned and may experience many different emotions from worry to anger. For some children there are underlying reasons why the child might actually want to avoid school, such as personal crises with other children, undiagnosed learning disabilities, anxiety about reading or performing for classmates, embarrassment in gym class, or fear that parental demands cannot be met.

When that is the case, continued school avoidance may actually reinforce headaches as a "successful" coping strategy on the child's part.

One method of encouraging increased functioning is called a *behavioral contract*. This contract is a written and signed agreement specifying an important change in behavior. Behavioral contracting can be very helpful in managing a variety of different pain-related behaviors. We have found it to be particularly helpful in encouraging children with difficult headache problems to return to school.

> Case Illustration A 12-year-old boy was brought to our center by his mother. He had daily headaches and had not attended school during the previous four weeks. Headaches were beginning in the morning before school or occurred shortly after his arrival. The boy described a seven-year history of sharp, pounding pressure over the right eye with nausea to the point of vomiting. During our session he described a history of panic reactions to pain, with associated negative thoughts such as "What am I going to do?" "What is this going to be like?" "Will it be a bad one?" "Where does it hurt right now?" "I've got to get rid of this headache" "I think a headache is going to start any time." He was so concerned that he might develop a headache at school and throw up in class that even the thought of returning to school created a great deal of anxiety. It appeared that school avoidance may have helped maintain this headache crisis, since the child never had an opportunity to fully test whether he could actually learn to tolerate some level of pain and remain in school.
>
> After a detailed discussion and an explanation of

"learned pain"—the idea of how avoidance behavior can maintain reactions of panic which may further fuel the headache itself—the child and his mother agreed to follow the behavioral contract (school attendance plan) shown in Table 9. The plan began with a small step selected by this young man—attending only one class period a day. It included an agreement to avoid talking about headache to decrease his attention to pain as well as a plan for dealing with questions from his friends. The plan also included a positive reinforcer selected by the youngster to help further motivate his school attendance.

Over the course of the next six weeks, he added more classes until he was once again in school on a full-time basis. He was warmly and enthusiastically praised for attending school "even with a bad headache." He also later reported changes in his thoughts from the earlier series of anxious questions to "I've got the headache but I can stand it." Two months after the first school attendance plan, his mother said that several teachers had told her son that his school behavior had dramatically improved. He received no preventive medication and stopped using any medication for acute pain by the third month of treatment. Although he received some biofeedback training, this was not started until he was attending school regularly three periods a day.

TABLE 9

A. Young Patient's Plan for School Attendance

1. Start with one period, no matter how you feel. The period will be reading class.

2. Stay *no longer* than one period.

3. Do not talk about how you feel during or after that period, whether you feel good or bad.

4. If someone asks how you feel, do not answer, or say "I don't want to talk about it."

5. When you have attended one period for five (5) days, your mother or father will take you to a target range, the next day if possible.

Signed

_____   _____
Child   Parent

                                             _____
                                             Psychologist

A one-year follow-up revealed that he was continuing to attend school regularly and missed only

two days in the preceding five months, experienced
only one episode of vomiting, and had headache-
free periods of up to three weeks' duration. He
used only aspirin occasionally for his headaches
and according to his mother continued with plans
and other activities whether he had a headache or
not.

Our experience with many other young people suggests
that similar plans must be put into effect as soon as reason-
ably possible. Lengthy delays increase the child's anxiety,
and it is often better to begin with a class period at the start
of the school day so that the child does not worry about
what will occur during the morning. Although the return to
school is non-negotiable, the child should be allowed some
influence over selecting which classes will be involved and
identifying reinforcers. Following the modified schoolday,
the child can return home and spend the rest of the day as
desired.

The central concept is the child's attendance *despite how
he or she feels*. This may at times be difficult, but it is
critical. Parents need to enthusiastically and frequently express their pride and pleasure, reinforced by physical affec-
tion with each day's attendance. Parents should avoid unnecessary discussion of the child's pain. In some cases,
complete avoidance of such discussions is necessary, while
in others a brief, structured discussion under limited circumstances once or twice a day and in defined periods of time
can be useful. The child can be asked to describe the degree
of pain, and the parents can express recognition and the
belief that things will soon be better. This planned discussion helps protect the child from feelings of neglect and the
parents from feelings of guilt.

Finally, the parents and the child should realize that even

with an open agreement about school attendance, there will be some increase in anxiety as the time for the actual school return approaches. In one case, a young man in our practice actually vomited outside the school door in anticipation of the return. When the mother called later to ask for guidance, she agreed with some encouragement to follow through with the plan the next day as originally worked out, even in the event of another crisis. Once the child made it past the initial fear and learned that he could actually tolerate being in school, the entire mood and outlook improved dramatically, and he was able to complete the full return within one week.

Summing Up

A detailed exploration of thoughts and behaviors related to headache and the patterns of antecedents and consequents of pain can be very helpful in developing an effective program for managing headache. Together with relaxation and biofeedback training this approach can allow the person in pain to take an active role in his or her care. Of course, biological triggers are very important in understanding headache, and medicine can be helpful and even necessary for some. However, an understanding and modification of headache-related thoughts and behaviors can be equally important and necessary for others.

17

Pain as a Cry for Help

Michael R. Barnat, Ph.D.,
and Joel R. Saper, M.D.

Not all pain causes suffering, and not all suffering is painful. Many persons may experience pain without a strong emotional and suffering attachment, while others suffer immensely at times when the pain is either minimal or diminishing. It is this interplay between the mind and the body that so tests all of us in our understanding of human nature and the way it expresses its agony and needs.

A person's report of pain may represent a "cry for help" for a variety of life problems. Unspoken distresses unsuccessfully addressed or resolved will frequently occur or recur as other problems, such as pain that is difficult to treat. Failure to identify and resolve these sources of personal desperation renders ineffective even the most appropriate forms of pain therapy.

The often complex problems of patients with chronic pain challenges the resourcefulness of physicians and other health care providers, requiring compassion and flexibility of thinking. Attitudes toward the patient and his or her reported distress will be a major determinant of the outcome of therapy. The following observations are designed to help the general public, as well as physicians, nurses, and other health care professionals working with pain patients to recognize certain special problems, resolve them when possible, and make appropriate referrals when necessary. The subjects addressed include recognizing psychological need, the ''pain patient'' and ''pain family,'' suicide and lethal behaviors, and the psychotic patient with headache and pain. A brief description of psychotherapy as it applies to patients like these is also included.

Recognizing Psychological Need

If a patient displays any of the following behaviors, the doctor or other health care professional will want to make a thorough exploration of the headache and pain patient's current life circumstances:
- Recurring visits to an emergency room.
- Insistence on narcotic or other pain-relieving medication.
- A pattern of paradoxical (opposite) responses to medication.
- Troubled family interactions.
- Angry or defiant behavior.
- Inappropriate mood.
- Conflicting messages or signals from the patient or a family member.

In short, if pain is and does not appear to be relieved by

otherwise appropriate treatment, psychological factors must be explored. If psychological factors are present, they must be confronted.

It is important for the care giver to be frank about his or her limitations. Few patients will resist compassionate exasperation expressed by their physician or health professional. Such openness may even put him or her into a more human perspective. If the care giver concludes that emotional problems are playing a critical role in the pain process, he or she should explain how this conclusion was arrived at. Honest confrontation in conventional language is a most important therapeutic tool. The more time that is spent to address these problems and the more forthright the presentation, the more effective will be the message. When a referral to a mental health specialist is made, there must be assurance that the referral does not reflect disinterest or imply punishment.

The Pain Patient and the Pain Family

Pain is an unavoidable but endurable part of life, and for most people acute pain or illness is a problem for which they are appropriately equipped to cope, at least temporarily; they have sufficient capacity to bind fear, obtain beneficial therapy, and solicit the appropriate responses from employer and family. When the symptom passes, normal functions are resumed.

When pain continues over a long period, however, resources can become quickly spent. The person is given to worry and doubt, and tolerance of family and employer dissipates. Over time, status changes from, in Dr. Richard Sternbach's words, the *patient in pain*, to *the pain patient*. For the pain patient, and by extension, the pain family, pain becomes the way of relating to others. Suffering becomes the central focus of life, bringing with it claims to money, compassion, time, care, and/or social respectability. It justifies failure and avoidance of responsibility, and discourages expectation. The pain patient cannot easily give up the claim once entrenched, nor are these dynamics likely to reverse spontaneously.

A number of underlying dynamics are possible explanations for these circumstances. Some families stay together solely because of the continued and chronic illness of one member; few or no other interests bind them. In other families, pain has become a form of political control: "I want you home at seven o'clock because I have a headache," (not because I care about you). In still other families ego competition exists. One family member openly takes pride and rejoices in stoicism, compared to another's complaining.

Members of the pain (headache) family knowingly or unknowingly encourage the patient's dependency or prolongation of illness. They act as enablers, allowing, out of guilt, sympathy or other feeling, demands to succeed and control. Thus, successful intervention must focus simultaneously on treatment for the symptom *and* on the family system in which it plays an important role. Professionals working with such problems are encouraged to explain the situation to the patient as they understand it. The therapist suggests, for example: "In a funny way, sometimes people in families need someone to be sick. That may be because when Dad is sick, then at least he is home and you get to see him."

The goal must be to encourage normal family functions and dynamics and to help the members distinguish their dependency on illness; reduce that portion of the family's income derived from or devoted to illness or medical expense, respectively; and assist the patient to find more constructive ways of coping with the challenges of family life.

Suicidal and Lethal Behaviors

Some of the most dramatic cries for help involve suicidal or destructive fantasies or behavior. Such fantasies are not uncommon as a reaction to chronic pain or in response to someone close to the patient who is perceived as unsympathetic and uncaring.

Ironically, the fleeting fantasy of death can play a survival role. A failed suicidal gesture may discharge built-up emotions and thus assist in the adjustment to unremitting pain. Self-destructive attempts may in a metaphorical way express an inability to establish boundaries to pain or depression. The suicidal fantasy indicates a feeling of helplessness and associated rage.

Self-destructive ideation may take the form of passing illusions or threats. It may occur in the form of repeated accidents, drug dependency, and overuse of symptomatic medications. Overindulgence and obesity can be suicidal intentions in disguise. For some depressed people the option or eventuality of suicide is assumed and does not require demonstration or verbalization. A care giver may easily overlook this potential.

A respectful inquiry into suicidal fantasies is appropriate. Some believe that opening these doors will convince an uncertain patient to consider suicide more seriously. Compassionate curiosity, however, greatly reduces this risk.

The conventional signs and indicators of suicidal risk include: a history of gestures (attempts or efforts at suicide), discussion of the fantasy, obsession with suicide, a family history of suicide, the sudden and unexplained elevation of mood in a seriously depressed person, the announcement "I am going to kill myself," or a sudden interest in finalizing one's affairs, such as drawing up a will.

Suicidal statements or efforts also have an important impact on families. They serve either to distance or to control the family members.

Psychotherapy

During therapy sessions, the patient and others are encouraged to talk about the pain problem as they experience it. The history of the symptom and the range of coping skills (religious values, philosophy, dependencies, and medication) are explored. This process, in addition to establishing the basis for the complaint, helps in the ventilation of fear and reduces anxiety. The psychotherapist may choose to explain the complex dynamics (interacting psychological influences) as these emerge and are demonstrated during the session.

The purpose of short-term psychotherapy is to focus upon the person more than on the pain itself. The goal is to discuss problems, not to "kill the pain."

Psychotherapy can be used to encourage patients to cooperate in a treatment plan, to resolve unrelated emotional or family problems, to help reduce the tension associated with pain, or to relieve the frustration of both patients and health care professionals. In addition, psychotherapy can support patients during crisis.

The outcome often depends on the contribution made by patients themselves. Some people have already achieved all but crucial insight into their own role in the pain problem and simply need confirmation of their thoughts. Others are still avoiding the thought of some personal responsibility.

Summing Up

For many kinds of health problems, self-reflection is not crucial. Some but not all headache and chronic pain patients possess a complex mosaic of personal, social, and physiological elements, and introspection may be helpful. Medication and education are mutually beneficial and increase the probability of improvement in cases of distress that is hard or difficult to relieve. A person's concerns about abandonment, labeling, debility, economic compensation, sexual impotence, harrassment at work, or the normal distresses of marriage, school, and parenthood will be interwoven with reports of unremitting pain. Some people will not dare discuss these problems with anyone unless their troubles are disguised as physical complaints. Hearing and accepting the person on his or her own terms (physical problem) but at the same time insisting upon a therapeutic direction and focus reduce anxiety and desperation and enhance the likelihood of a beneficial outcome.

18

Drug Overuse Among Those With Headaches

Very often it is necessary for people who suffer from recurring headaches as well as health care professionals treating people with pain to confront a serious drug overuse problem. The extent of this problem is difficult to judge. At our center, the Michigan Headache and Neurological Institute, we estimate that at least half the patients seeking our help for headaches indulge in excessive use of medications to relieve their distress. It is not unusual for first-time patients to report the consumption of 10 to 30 simple pain-relieving tablets per day, 6 to 8 mg of ergotamine tartrate daily, or the regular ingestion of large amounts of tranquilizing, hypnotic, or narcotic analgesics.

Obtaining an accurate history of this overuse is difficult.

Some patients are ashamed of their reliance on drugs. Others may be frightened that their medications will be taken away if they admit to the extent of their use. Some believe that only prescription medications need be reported and thus refrain from discussing their use of over-the-counter (OTC) pain remedies.

There are no generally accepted standards for establishing that abuse is present. The following informal criteria are presented as guidelines.

- Daily or almost daily use of analgesics.
- Recurring use of 10 mg or more of ergotamine tartrate or its derivatives per week.
- Every day, every other day, or every third day use of ergotamine tartrate.
- Daily or almost daily use of compounds containing barbiturates and other sedative or tranquilizing substances.

Among the specific questions your physician may ask are:

- How long will 50 aspirin last?
- Are you buying pain remedies in large amounts?
- Do you always carry medications with you?
- Do you keep them in strategic locations around your house, office, or car?
- Do you take the medications ritualistically, that is, automatically when you awake or retire or other times of the day?

Pain-Relieving Drugs and Compounds

Nonnarcotic pain-relieving drugs may be obtained by simple purchase or by prescription. Most contain aspirin or acetaminophen, or both. Many are combinations of these agents, plus caffeine. The so-called "sinus headache medications" combine these agents with antihistamines and mild decongestants. Table 4, pages 70–71, lists the ingredients of common non-prescription drugs. Table 10 lists some prescription drugs and their nonprescription components.

Aspirin, acetaminophen, and caffeine accumulate in kidney tissue. They may have a cumulative damaging effect on kidney tissue. Many prescription compounds also contain barbiturates or codeine. Propoxyphene (Darvon) and other agents may also be combined with simple analgesics. Aside from the potential risks imposed by these combinations, persons with allergic responses to one or more of the contained substances (such as aspirin) may not be aware of their presence in medications sold over the counter or prescribed as combinations.

Combinations containing aspirin, acetaminophen, and caffeine may have no greater effectiveness than simple aspirin. Sedative components, though adding a dimension to therapy, generally do not offer increased pain relief but impose the added risk of addiction and withdrawal.

Aspirin Aspirin, of which an estimated 50 million pounds are consumed yearly in the United States, is well known for its beneficial effects in relieving pain, fever, and inflammation. It also has an anticlotting effect. This discussion focuses on aspirin's harmful implications when overused.

The most commonly reported symptom of importance from aspirin use is minor gastrointestinal upset. Two to ten percent of people taking aspirin occasionally experience minor distress. An estimated 30 to 50% of patients taking excessive aspirin (ten tablets a day or more) experience marked gastric upset. Aspirin may directly irritate the mucous membranes that line the digestive tract.

TABLE 10

Active Ingredients in Some Prescription Analgesics

Drug	Aspirin	Acetamino-phen
Darvocet-N 50	—	325
Darvocet-N 100	—	650
Darvon	—	
Darvon-N	—	
Darvon Compound	389 mg	—
Darvon Compound-65	389 mg	—
Demerol	—	
Dilaudid	—	
Empirin	325 mg	—
Fiorinal	325 mg	—
Micrainin	325 mg	—
Percocet	—	325
Percodan	325	—
Phenaphen	—	325
Synalgos-DC	356.4	—
Tylenol with codeine	300	—
Tylox	—	500
Vicodin	—	500

Caffeine	Available With Codeine	Other
—	—	50 mg propoxyphene napsylate
—	—	100 mg propoxyphene napsylate
—	—	32 or 65 mg propoxyphene HCl
—	—	100 mg propoxyphene napsylate
32.4	—	32 mg propoxyphene HCl
32.4	—	65 mg propoxyphene HCl
—	—	50 or 100 mg meperidine HCl
—	—	1 to 4 mg hydromorphone HCl
—	yes	—
40	yes	50 mg butalbital
—	—	200 mg meprobamate
—	—	5 mg oxycodone HCl
—	—	4.5 mg oxycodone HCl
		0.38 mg oxycodone terephthalate
—	yes	—
30	—	16 mg dihydrocodeine bitartrate
—	yes	—
—	—	4.5 mg oxycodone HCl
		0.38 mg oxycodone terephthalate
		5 mg hydrocodone bitartrate

Invisible (occult) blood is present in the stool of most patients taking moderate to high dosages of aspirin. This effect is especially important in women who regularly have heavy blood flow during menstruation. It is estimated that six to eight aspirin tablets a day will result in the loss of one-half to one teaspoon in the stool. Greater daily intake can cause 6 teaspoons or more of blood loss per day. Over two-thirds of patients regularly overusing aspirin have reduced red blood cell production.

Patients sensitive to aspirin may also be sensitive to salicin-containing foods, which include apples, oranges, and bananas. Processed foods and medications containing tartrazine dye or sodium benzoate, and iodide-containing agents may also induce a reaction. Patients with aspirin sensitivity may also react adversely to drugs containing nonsteroidal anti-inflammatory agents, including Nuprin, Advil, and other nonprescription drugs.

Aspirin is truly one of the miracle drugs. It is an effective and relatively safe painkiller, may reduce the risk of heart attack and stroke in low daily dosage (less than one adult tablet per day), reduces fever, and is important in arthritis conditions. But, in excessive amounts, or in certain patients, aspirin can be dangerous. Moreover, daily use in patients with headache may make headaches worse because of the rebound action we discussed earlier.

Acetaminophen Several OTC and prescribed analgesics contain aspirin or acetaminophen, alone or in combination. Acetaminophen relieves pain and fever but does not reduce inflammation.

Excessive use of acetaminophen may affect kidney or liver function. Like aspirin, acetaminophen is an important and effective pain reliever, but excessive or daily use is troublesome.

Caffeine Most pain-relieving combinations contain caffeine. Some reports suggest that caffeine improves pain relief, exerts a favorable influence on mood, and enhances intestinal absorption of ergotamine and other substances. Other studies do not substantiate these claims.

Caffeine has an interesting history. Once referred to as "the devil's brew," a "loathesome poison," and "the nectar of the gods," it was the central theme of Bach's *Coffee Contata*, Bach's response to Frederick the Great's 1732 proposed ban on caffeine.

Legends abound. In one, a tired Chinese Buddhist monk fell asleep during a nine-year meditation. Awakening, he impulsively cut off his eyelashes in order to guarantee no recurrence of his sinful behavior. His severed lashes fell to the ground, sprouted tea, and provided a drink capable of banishing sleep. The first coffee break was alleged to have occurred when a shepherd named Kaldi (circa A.D. 850) witnessed his goats acting strangely after eating berries from a nearby shrub. The shepherd sampled these and experienced a stimulant effect, later ascribed to caffeine.

The mental changes of caffeine were indirectly acknowledged by the *London Public Advisor*, in a story dated January 27, 1774, when it was reported that "...400 or 500 chests of tea have so contaminated the water of Boston Harbor that the fish may have contracted a disorder not unlike the nervous complaints of the body."

Caffeine is a stimulant and has many effects on the body, including an influence on the heart, lungs, blood vessels, muscles, secretion of stomach acid, urinary and kidney function, and metabolism. The stimulant effect of caffeine may be followed by depression after a while or when discontinued.

Caffeine can be fatal in large doses (10 grams or more). Unwanted reactions occur following ingestion of approximately 1 gram (8 to 10 cups of brewed coffee). These include insomnia, restlessness and excitement, ringing in the ears, disturbances of vision, tremors, rapid heartbeat and palpitations, increased urination, and rapid breathing. Most persons ingesting large dosages of caffeine daily do not experience toxic symptoms for years. For most adults, 300 to 400 mg of caffeine per day represents an excessive load. Adaptation may develop, however, and chronic use of 900 mg or more, approximately equivalent to nine cups of coffee per day, is common. Blood levels peak within 30 to 45 minutes after oral ingestion.

Table 11 lists the amount of caffeine in major sources. Refer to Table 12 for the amount of caffeine in popular drug combinations.

The symptoms of caffeinism are divided into those of mood disturbances, sleep disturbances, and withdrawal. The mood disturbances associated with caffeine usage include anxiety and related complaints such as jitteriness, tremulousness, agitation, irritability, muscle twitching, lightheadedness, palpitations, and gastrointestinal distress. Dr. John Greden of the University of Michigan has reported several patients initially diagnosed as suffering from anxiety neurosis who were instead experiencing caffeine intoxication.

Sleep disturbances include delayed sleep onset and more frequent nighttime awakening. Caffeine counteracts the sedatives and tranquilizers, leading to some increased need and dependence on medications. Withdrawal symptoms from caffeine excess include headache, grogginess, and malaise. Drowsiness, lethargy, runny nose, yawning, irritability, depression, and even nausea may be present.

TABLE 11

Caffeine in Food Sources

	Estimated Caffeine (mg)
Brewed coffee/cup	100–150
Instant coffee/cup	85–100
Tea/cup	60–75
Decaffeinated coffee/cup	2–4
Cola (8 oz)	40–60
Cocoa/cup	40–55
Chocolate bar	25

TABLE 12

Caffeine in Common Drugs

Drug	mg	Drug	mg
APC	32	Anacin	32
Cafergot	100	Bromoseltzer	32
Darvon compound	32	Cope	32
Fiorinal	40	Midol	32
Wigraine	100	Vanquish	60
		Excedrin	66
		Pre-mens	30

Headaches associated with caffeine use can occur as a consequence of too much caffeine or to withdrawal. The caffeine withdrawal headache occurs 8 to 16 hours after the last ingestion in a person who is consuming excessive amounts. It is characterized as generalized and throbbing discomfort, usually occurring in the morning upon awakening and promptly relieved by more caffeine. Accompanying symptoms include fatigue, grogginess, clouded thinking, and loss of ambition. (Many headache conditions are present upon awakening and headache patients are known to take abundant amounts of caffeine, thus confusing the issue.)

Regular and excessive users of caffeine-containing substances, when compared to those using much lesser amounts, demonstrated elevated muscle tension levels and other anxiety elements three or more hours following sudden discontinuance, suggesting that anxiety symptoms may be a consequence of both toxicity to caffeine and withdrawal from it.

Consequences of Analgesic Overuse

There are many additional body symptoms that can come from taking too many painkillers, not the least of which is the possible increase in intensity and frequency of the pain. If painkillers contain sedative medication, mental changes caused by too much medication may be followed by hyperactivity and even seizures upon discontinuance. Tremors, increased pain, muscle cramps, insomnia, agitation, and other symptoms are quite common in such a setting. In addition to all of this, medications that might otherwise prevent headache appear not to be effective, or as effective, when given to patients who take painkillers daily. Discontinuance of excessive analgesic usage may bring about a dramatic improvement in pain, though pain may first intensify for a time immediately following discontinuance.

Ergot Overuse

Ergotamine is derived from a fungus of rye and other grains. Epidemics of gangrene and mental changes due to contaminated rye were reported in the literature as early as 1670. More recent outbreaks have been documented in Russia (1926), Ireland (1929), and France (1953). In an article entitled *A Satan Loose in Salem*, ergot intoxication was incriminated as the cause of mental aberrations responsible for bizarre behavior ascribed to witchery.

Ergotamine's usefulness in the treatment of migraine-type headaches was first recognized in 1883. Ergotamines have many effects on body function and influence blood vessels (generally producing constriction). They also affect the brain and other organ systems. They may delay the emptying of the stomach, may damage the lining of blood vessels, and may cause contraction of the uterus, a fact that has resulted in the use of excessive amounts of this medication to induce (very dangerously) abortions.

Despite the wide and often excessive use of these agents, severe reactions including dangerous constriction of blood vessels and reduction of blood flow to the organs is relatively rare. Some patients seem more susceptible to these side effects than others. Among the other symptoms of excessive use of ergot medications are mental changes including confusion and mood disturbances, epileptic seizures, severe muscle cramps, changes in vision, disturbances of temperature regulation, reduction of blood flow to most organs including the brain, and damage to blood vessels.

During the past several years, increasing attention has been paid to the likelihood that frequent use of ergotamine medication may result in a self-sustaining headache/medication cycle resulting from addiction to the drug. This problem appears to stem from a dependency that develops over time and which is very subtle and easily overlooked by physicians. It is characterized by recurring headaches accompanied by the irresistible and regular use of ergotamine, which appears to be the only effective medicine to relieve the headache. Patients caught in this cycle frequently take the drug at least three times per week and usually more often. Preventive medications will not be effective until withdrawal from ergotamine takes place. This problem develops on a background of occasional, effective, and appropriate use of ergotamine, but over time an escalation of headache frequency and drug use occurs. It is strongly recommended that patients using ergotamine limit their use to *no more than once or twice per week*. If more is needed, a change in treatments is required.

It must be emphasized that ergotamine tartrate is one of the most effective and useful agents for treating severe migraine. Its use has brought about meaningful control for headaches in patients who otherwise would not benefit from modern therapy. However, when ergotamine is used, it must be used in patients who can take the drug safely and with limitations on frequency and total dosage. As with all other medications, inappropriate usage can be hazardous.

Summing Up

The headache patient who overuses medications presents a special challenge. Personal experience over several years prompts me to conclude that most overusers need to be admitted to the hospital at first. There, efforts directed at reducing the offending medications and addressing the many additional physical and emotional needs can be more adequately carried out. Hospitalization in a special headache unit provides an opportunity to carefully discontinue the drugs, to attend to the consequences of overuse, and to develop the appropriate treatment programs. It also gives physician and patient time to confront issues that may critically influence the pain syndrome and serve to aggravate the biological predisposition considered basic in many chronic headache disorders.

Between 1978 and 1980, we developed what was at that time the first inpatient specialty headache unit in a hospital for many of our patients who had daily and otherwise untreatable headaches, frequently accompanied by severe drug overuse problems. As the unit grew, it began to attract patients from all over the world, We added additional programs including intensive education seminars, individual therapy, self-help programs, exercise and programs for stopping smoking, and many other program components. Patients generally remain in the hospital for approximately 10 to 14 days and receive regular medical care in addition to the other treatment elements. The successful results that we have achieved in many patients who have not otherwise received benefits has been gratifying, although for reasons not fully understood, not all patients will get better. Currently, over 75% of patients who have not been helped by other treatment interventions appear to respond to this type of aggressive and intensive treatment program.

This chapter has focused on the possible consequences of the excessive use of some of the medications used to treat pain, particularly headache. The overuse problem is widespread because of the desperate nature of many headache problems and because effective treatments have not been made available. In addition, advertisements which promote "quick cures" have added greatly to the problem. Many individuals with headache will awaken each morning in pain and retire with it each night. Many have sought out various medical as well as nonmedical avenues of help, ranging from qualified health care to nonqualified sources that offer simple explanations and "miracle" therapies. Many individuals have turned to painkillers just to "get through the day." Marital, work, and other relationships suffer as the quality of life deteriorates.

The use of painkillers can be an important component of a good treatment program, but limitations must be employed. With proper restriction and wise administration, analgesics may temporarily relieve pain. Many of the over-the-counter as well as prescription analgesics offer an important controlling method. But inappropriate and excessive use can be seriously harmful.

A Concluding Word

Chronic and recurring headache can promote feelings of desperation and loneliness in its sufferers. Emotional, marital, and socioeconomic distress are common. Headache disorders themselves are not completely understood, but in the past few years, research and clinical work have brought major breakthroughs in our capacity to help patients afflicted with this disorder.

It seems likely that most patients with recurring headache are biologically different from those who appear to have similar life-styles, personalities, psychological stresses, and medical backgrounds, but who do not suffer recurring headache. Subtle changes in brain or blood vessel function will probably be more clearly understood in the next several years. At this time, however, important links to our understanding are missing.

Despite these limitations, current treatment approaches and other efforts outlined in this book can bring relief for most people who suffer from these conditions. Specialty centers have sprouted throughout the country, and as mentioned earlier, special units in hospitals have begun to take on the task of treating the most difficult headache problems. In our center, we estimated that over 75% of patients, many of whom have been referred to us from around the world, show major improvement in headache control and are able to overcome the devastation and desperation that can accompany severe and often daily pain. Unfortunately, not all people are satisfactorily helped. For some, it is because their condition exceeds current knowledge. For others, deepseated psychological issues can defeat even the most committed effort by those from whom help is sought.

Nevertheless, isolation and despair are no longer appropriate sentiments. Discrimination against those with headaches, based upon misunderstanding, myth, and prejudice, should not be tolerated. Patients suffering from chronic recurring headaches can and must demand the same respect, time, and committed effort directed at their condition as are accorded other and at times less troublesome medical illnesses. Current treatment techniques have changed the outlook, and effective control over headaches should be expected for those who make a serious effort at finding the right professional to help them and who cooperate fully in their treatment regimen.

To those of you who suffer from this condition or have family or loved ones who do, many of us are working hard to help overcome the problem. Never give up!

—J.R.S.

References

Bakal, D.A., Demjen S., and Kaganov, J.A. 1981. Cognitive behavioral treatment of chronic headache. *Headache*, *21*:81–86.

Barnat, M.R., and Lake, A.E. III. 1983. Patient attitudes about headache. *Headache*, *23*:229–237.

Basmajian, J.V., (Ed.). *Biofeedback: Principles and Practice for Clinicians*. Baltimore: Williams and Wilkins. Second Edition.

Blanchard, E.B., Andrasik, F., Ahles, T.A., et al. 1980. Migraine and Tension Headache: A meta-analytic review. *Behavior Therapy*, *11*:613–631.

Blanchard, E.B., Andrasik, F., Neff, D.F., et al. 1982. Biofeedback and relaxation training with three kinds of headache: Treatment effects and their prediction. *Journal of Consulting and Clinical Psychology, 50*:562–575.

Blanchard, E.B., Jaccard, J., Andrasik, F., et al. 1985. Reduction in headache patient's medical expenses associated with biofeedback and relaxation treatments. *Biofeedback and Self-Regulation, 10*:63–68.

Claghorn, J.L., Mathew, R.J., Largen, J.W., et al. 1981. Directional effects of skin temperature self-regulation on regional cerebral blood flow on normal subjects and migraine patients. *American Journal of Psychiatry, 138*:1182–1187.

Dalessio, D. F. 1980. *Wolff's Headache*. New York: Oxford University Press.

Holroyd, K.A., Penzien, D.B., Hursey, K.G., et al. 1984. Change mechanisms in EMG Biofeedback Training: Cognitive changes underlying improvements in tension headache. *Journal of Consulting and Clinical Psychology, 52*:1039–1053.

Kudrow, L. 1980. *Cluster Headache*. New York: Oxford University Press.

Lake, A.E. III, and Pingel, J.D. 1983. Long-term follow-up of biofeedback effectiveness for patients with mixed migraine–muscle contraction headache. Presented at the 25th Annual Meeting of the American Association for the Study of Headache. Toronto, Canada.

Lake, A.E. III, and Pingel, J.D. 1984. Positive and negative side effects related to biofeedback–assisted relaxation training for headache. Presented at the 26th Annual Meeting of the American Association for the Study of Headache. San Francisco, California.

Lance, J. W. 1982. *Mechanism and Management of Headache*. 4th edition. London: Butterworth Scientific Press.

Libo, L.M., and Arnold, G.E. 1983. Does training to criteria influence improvement? A follow-up study of

EMG and thermal biofeedback. *Journal of Behavioral Medicine,* *6*:397–404.

Mathew, N. T. 1981. Prophylaxis of migraine and mixed headache: A randomized control study. *Headache, 21*:105–109.

Mathew, N. T., Stubits, E., and Nigam, M. 1982. Transformation of migraine into daily headache: Analysis of factors. *Headache, 22*:66–68.

Rapoport, A. 1986. Analgesic rebound. *Topics in Pain Management, 1*(8):29–32.

Rapoport, A., Weeks, R.E., Sheftell, F. D., et al. 1986. The "analgesic washout period": A critical variable in the evaluation of headache treatment efficacy. Abstract. *Neurology* [Supplement], *36*:100–101.

Raskin, N. H., and Appenzeller, O. 1980. *Headache.* Philadelphia: W. B. Saunders.

Raskin, N. H., and Schwartz, R. K. 1980. Interval therapy of migraine: Long-term results. *Headache, 20*:336–340.

Saper, J. R. 1986. Changing perspectives on chronic headache. *Clinical Journal of Pain Management, 2*:19–28.

Saper, J. R. 1983. *Headache Disorders: Current Concepts and Treatment Strategies.* Littleton, Massachusetts: Wright PSG.

Saper, J. R. 1985–1986. *Topics in Pain Management,* Volumes 1 and 2.

Saper, J. R., Johnson, T., and Van Meter, M. 1983. "Mixed headache": A chronic headache complex. A study of 500 patients. Abstract. *Headache, 23*:143.

Saper, J. R., and Jones, J. M. 1986. Ergotamine tartrate dependency: Features and possible mechanisms. *Clinical Neuropharmacology, 9*(3):244–256.

Turk, D.C., Meichenbaum, D., and Genest, M. 1983. *Pain and Behavioral Medicine: A cognitive–behavioral perspective.* New York: Guilford Press.

Suggested Reading and Self-Help Books

Benson, H. 1984. *Beyond the Relaxation Response*. New York: Berkeley.

Brown, B.B. 1977. *Biofeedback and the Art of Biofeedback*. New York: Bantam.

Burns, D.D. 1980. *Feeling good: The new mood therapy*. New York: Signet.

Davis, M., Eschelman, E.R., and McKay, M. 1980. *The Relaxation and Stress Reduction Workbook*. Richmond, CA: New Harbinger.

Fensterheim, H. and Baer, J. 1975. *Don't Say Yes When You Want to Say No*. New York: Dell.

Friedman, M. and Ulmer, D. 1984. *Treating Type A Behavior — and Your Heart*. New York: Fawcett Crest.

Girdano, D.A. and Everly, G.S. 1979. *Controlling Stress and Tension: A Holistic Approach*. Englewood Cliffs, New Jersey: Prentice-Hall.

McKay, M., Davis, M., and Fanning, P. 1981. *Thoughts and Feelings: The Art of Cognitive Stress Intervention*. Richmond, CA: New Harbinger.

Index

157

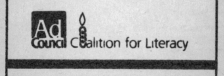